Dedication

To my incredible wife,

Your unwavering belief in me and your constant support have been my greatest sources of strength.

This book is as much yours as it is mine, for without your love, help and encouragement, it would never have been possible.

Thank you for always believing in me, even when I doubted myself.

With all my love,

David

Contents

Disclaimer

The information presented in this book is based on my personal experiences managing and overcoming IBS over the span of 12 years. I am not a medical professional, and this book should not be seen as a substitute for professional medical advice, diagnosis, or treatment.

Before making any changes to your diet, lifestyle, or treatment plan, please consult your GP or a qualified healthcare provider. It is crucial to follow the guidance of your healthcare provider and to continue taking any prescribed medications unless advised otherwise by your doctor.

IBS can vary greatly among individuals, and what worked for me may not be suitable for everyone. Use this book as a guide alongside professional support to find the best approach for your unique situation.

Preface

When I first began struggling with IBS, I was met with a mix of confusion, embarrassment, and frustration. IBS isn't just an uncomfortable inconvenience; it can affect nearly every part of your life—what you eat, where you go, how you feel, and even what you believe is possible for yourself. This book is a testament to the journey from living in that discomfort to finding peace and control over your body and mind.

I wrote *The IBS Escape Plan* as both a guide and a companion for those on this journey. This isn't just a collection of tips; it's a holistic approach to managing IBS, rooted in years of my own experience. This book is divided into two essential parts: the **Internal World**, which focuses on mindset, emotional responses, and stress perception, and the **External World**, which addresses diet, lifestyle, and environmental factors. Together, they form a complete view of IBS management that goes beyond symptom relief and seeks to empower readers to live fully, despite their condition.

Throughout these chapters, you'll come across "Tips"—essential reminders of actions you can take, which I've placed strategically to encourage real change. These are not demanding "rules" but rather practical suggestions that I hope will help you build confidence in your daily routines. Additionally, each chapter includes a Reflection and Practical Step section. This might be the most important part of the book because it invites you to reflect and actively apply what you've learned. There's no point in simply reading this book from cover to cover without taking action—I know because I've been there. I was once a self-help book junkie, always reading, feeling motivated, but never quite taking the leap to actually implement the ideas. I'd read one book and, rather than taking action, I'd move straight on to the next, feeding a cycle that felt good in the moment but ultimately didn't help.

To make the most of these reflections and practical steps, **I recommend getting a dedicated journal or notebook.** Use it to record your responses to prompts, track your experiences with the low-FODMAP diet, and note any specific triggers that come up along the way. This space will become a valuable tool for self-discovery and accountability as you progress.

This book isn't about motivation alone; it's about change, and real change requires action.

To illustrate, here's a story my dad told me **countless** times—a story that has stuck with me: "If there are five frogs by the side of a pond, and three decide to jump in, how many are left?" The answer: five! Even though they decided to jump, none of them actually did. My dad drilled this story into me, and although I may not have appreciated it back then, it's a powerful reminder that decisions alone don't create progress—taking action does. I hope this story serves as a reminder to engage fully with the exercises and tips in this book and not just decide to make changes but actually follow through.

What you'll find here is not a one-size-fits-all solution but rather a toolkit to help you understand your own triggers, whether they stem from within or from external influences. The journey through this book mirrors my own, and I've filled it with practical strategies and hard-earned wisdom that I hope will make your journey smoother.

For those of you reading this with the familiar discomfort of IBS, I want you to know that you're not alone. You're seen, understood, and capable of reclaiming control over your health. Relief, calm, and confidence are within reach, and my hope is that this book will serve as a roadmap for achieving them.

If your symptoms are severe and you're seeking immediate relief, you might consider reading Chapter 12, page 313, on diet first. Starting with dietary adjustments can provide some initial control over symptoms, making it easier to focus on other techniques as you read the rest of the book. However, I encourage you to approach the full journey with patience, as IBS management involves multiple factors, both physical and mental, that work together for lasting relief.

As you read, keep an open mind, engage fully with the techniques, and remember that progress often comes with small, consistent steps. This book is designed to empower you to make choices that support your well-being, and I encourage you to approach it with patience and self-compassion.

And now, I'd like to share the moment that sparked this journey—a story that stays with me to this day. It all began on a crowded bus in Korea:

Sitting at the back of a crowded bus packed with commuters, I was on my way to work, and they had already started. The dreaded stomach cramps.

"At least I have a seat", I thought to myself.

"Only 20 minutes longer and you'll be at work, it'll be okay. It WILL be okay".

It wasn't okay. The cramps got worse, and the idea of what was going to happen loomed over me—just the kind of thought that may cross the mind of anyone suffering from bowel-related problems. The worst possible scenario. I was going to shit myself, at the back of a bus, in a foreign country, and it's not even 8 am yet.

I clenched harder but as I did the feeling for release became stronger. That desperate release everyone has from time to time. Only here, I was stuck and with not much of a choice. Sweat was literally dripping off my face on this cool but unfortunate autumn morning in South Korea. I didn't think, so I just acted instinctively, as any sane human would, who was about to defecate while travelling on public transportation.

"Stop the bus!!" I screamed.

The driver, naturally, refused since we were on the motorway.

So I scrambled my way to the front and although I can't fully recall what I said exactly at that time it was along the lines of " I'm going to die!!" or "I need to go to the hospital!!" He reluctantly agreed when he saw my desperate, pitiful face and stopped on the hard shoulder. I got off.

"Bush...bush...where's a bush or a tree or a place no one will see me?"

I waited for the bus to leave. Dark thoughts and vivid images appeared in my mind of becoming a viral sensation on the internet. 'Brit abroad takes a shit on the side of the road', the caption would read. Several YouTubers would monetise my misery while the viewers would laugh with tears of schadenfreude.[1] It would be my 3 minutes of fame.

I just decided to walk slowly but surely and clearly like someone who was going to 'let it all out' so to speak. I had a strong sense of eyes watching me, my every move. Possibly a few cameras. Who was this foreigner? What on earth is he going to do? The tension in the air and clearly in my bowel were insurmountable.

If you are yet to have experienced anything similar to this, then I envy you, and if you have, I can only say I'm truly sorry to hear that you went through that. The aim of this book is to act as a guide to show you where I started - at the back of that dreaded bus many years ago and to today where I'm free, healthy and living life to the fullest. The

---

1. Schadenfreude (from German, meaning "harm-joy") refers to the pleasure derived from another person's misfortune.

journey, however, took 10 years. If any of the mistakes I learned from are helpful to you at all, then I'll be pleased that I wrote this book.

But, I know what you're thinking. "How did the damn story finish?" "Did you shit yourself?" "What the hell happened?" Well, for now, I'll just say don't bother searching on YouTube for it just yet. One of the bits of advice in the book is as follows:

It's not what happens to us which is important but what labels we give to situations in our lives which shape our thoughts and ultimately our reality.

In other words, the event doesn't affect you, the story you attach to it does.

But I didn't give up. This was the start of an 8-year journey to finding peace with my body. And I want to show you how you can do it too.

I hope you enjoy the book and I wish you all the best.

Now get ready for your journey.

Tips

Introduction

Understanding IBS and Your Journey

In recent years, the diagnosis of Irritable Bowel Syndrome (IBS) has undergone a major shift. It's no longer just considered a functional gastrointestinal disorder—now it's recognised as a disorder of gut-brain interaction (DGBI). This change reflects a deeper understanding of how IBS works: it's not just about an upset stomach or a bit of gut trouble. IBS happens because of dysfunctions in the communication between your gut and your brain. Stress, emotions, and even psychological factors can trigger physical symptoms in your gut, and gut issues can, in turn, make you feel more anxious or down. It's a two-way street!

For some, the causes of IBS might be a 50/50 mix of both internal and external factors—like two sides of the same coin. Your mindset and environment might play equal roles in shaping your symptoms. For others, IBS might be driven by what's happening inside—how you react to stress, anxiety, or even your own thoughts. Your gut is in constant conversation with your mind, and getting to grips with that can be a real eye-opener. But for some of you, IBS may be triggered more by external factors—whether it's the foods you eat, your lifestyle choices, allergies, or sensitivities like gluten or too much fibre. The more you understand what sets off your symptoms, the more empowered you'll feel to take control of your health.

That's exactly why I decided to split this book into two worlds: the Internal World and the External World. It's not just about what you eat or how you think—it's about how these two forces work together to impact your gut health. When you understand this connection, you'll be able to craft a more personalised, holistic plan for managing your IBS, one that addresses your life as a whole, rather than just focusing on symptoms.

The **Internal World** includes your mindset, thinking patterns, and perception of stress. Essentially, your thoughts and feelings shape the reality you create in your mind every day. If you're constantly anticipating the worst or holding on to anxiety, that internal state can directly influence how your body reacts, including your gut. The chapters in this section will help you reframe your thoughts, build resilience, and find mental strategies to soothe your symptoms.

The **External World** consists of the things outside of your mind that impact your well-being: your relationships, work, lifestyle choices, sleep patterns, diet, medication, and the objective stressors you face daily. Understanding how these factors play a role in your IBS is key to finding solutions. You'll learn how to make changes in your environment, diet, and daily habits to support a calmer gut and a more balanced life.

In this book, we'll look into how these two worlds intertwine, often in ways you haven't yet considered. Managing IBS isn't about a "one-size-fits-all" solution; it's about understanding the unique ways your internal and external worlds collide and impact your gut. As we explore both sides, you'll discover a clearer roadmap to managing your symptoms and keeping flare-ups at bay. Along the way, I'll share my own experiences—what's worked for me, what hasn't—and practical strategies that will help you take back control of your life, so that your gut doesn't dictate your every move.

Part 1

The Internal World

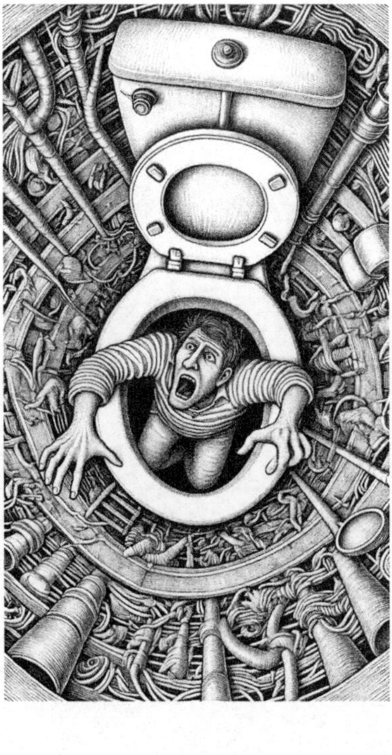

Chapter 1

IBS in Society

When you have a toothache, you go to the dentist. They'll find the problem and either pull your tooth or remove the decay, all with the ease of local anaesthetic. You break your leg, you're given a cast. You cut your finger, you get a plaster (or band-aid if you're American). These are straightforward solutions to obvious problems.

But what happens when your body gives you a more complicated message—when the symptoms aren't so easy to pin down? That's the confusion many people face with Irritable Bowel Syndrome (IBS). The first problem with IBS is that it isn't as straightforward as a broken bone or a toothache. There's no one pill, cast, or quick fix.

In 2012, I found myself moving to South Korea, ready to teach English to middle school students. After a peaceful year prior, teaching in a small French village, I anticipated another relaxing experience, immersed in a new culture, exploring, and bonding with my students. But my reality turned out to be far from that. I wasn't prepared for the chaos of disciplining unruly teens, dealing with kids sneaking cigarettes in the bathroom, or adjusting to a completely new language and way of life—all without much support from the staff.

Unsurprisingly, the stress of the situation began taking its toll. While I had dealt with some stomach issues before, they were never so severe that I thought much of them. However, within weeks of settling into my new job, my gut had a different plan. That's when the real symptoms of IBS hit—sharp abdominal pain, uncomfortable bloating, constant gas, and an aggravating cycle of diarrhoea and constipation. It felt like my body was fighting against me at every turn, and the stress only made things worse.

I tried everything I could to get things back to normal. Bland foods? Check. Bottled water? Check. Skipping meals entirely? Check, unfortunately. I even lost a significant amount of weight, hoping it might make a difference. But despite all my attempts to self-treat, nothing seemed to work. Looking back, I realise how much I didn't know at the time, and though my journey to getting a proper diagnosis was long and confusing, it led to a crucial turning point in my life.

***

The Turning Point

There was one day in particular that I'll never forget. The stress of managing unruly teenagers had reached its peak. I had barely eaten all day because I was terrified that food would trigger my symptoms. Yet,

I was still running out of the classroom frequently to go to the toilet. And by the time I got home, my gut was in knots, and I sat on my bed, clutching my stomach, feeling completely helpless. It became clear to me at that moment that I couldn't live like this—constantly fearing my own body's reactions.

***

Finding a Way Forward

That was when I decided to take a different approach. I started experimenting with small, controlled meals and gradually reintroducing foods in a way that didn't overwhelm my system. At first, I avoided anything that seemed risky—spicy foods, coffee, greasy foods and heavy meals were off the table. Instead, I stuck with bland, safe options like boiled chicken, rice, and cooked vegetables. Slowly, I would reintroduce foods in small portions, one by one, paying close attention to how my body reacted. For example, while yoghurt seemed manageable in small amounts, anything more would trigger my symptoms. Later on, I would find out about the now-popular low-FODMAP diet. It was a slow process, but I began to realise that it wasn't just about avoiding certain foods, but also about eating in a calm, mindful state and using relaxation techniques.

I started practising these techniques like rhythmic breathing, grounding, visualisation and reframing my negative automatic thoughts before work each day. It wasn't an overnight fix for sure—nothing ever is—but over time, I found that managing my stress helped ease the intensity of my symptoms. IBS didn't disappear, but I learned to manage how I responded to stress, and that made all the difference.

The thing about IBS is, it doesn't just affect your body. It takes a toll on your mental and emotional well-being, too. You feel isolated, frustrated, and, worst of all, powerless. There's no easy answer, no clear-cut solution. You're left wondering: Why me? What did I do to deserve this?

The truth is, IBS is a complex disorder that varies from person to person. What works for one person might not work for another. And to make matters worse, nobody truly knows what exactly causes it.

In my case, the stress of moving to a new country, adjusting to a new job, and dealing with a language barrier were all massive triggers. The physical discomfort was worsened by my emotional and psychological stress. The chaos in my life seemed to translate directly into chaos in my gut.

Irritable Bowel Syndrome (IBS) doesn't just exist in the body—it lives in the space between your brain and your gut, in the way stress affects your digestion, and in how you perceive and react to those stressors. This is where the mind-body connection comes into play, and why understanding this connection is so vital in managing IBS.

Tip #1: Get Tested at a Hospital

One of the first things you need to do if you think you might have IBS is to rule out any other potential causes of your symptoms. This means getting tested at a hospital or with a healthcare professional. While IBS doesn't have a single definitive test, it's important to ensure that nothing more serious is going on, for example Irritable Bowel Disease (IBD), Celiac disease or SIBO[1]

***

Understanding the Diagnosis

Even if you think you know what's going on with your body, it's always best to get a professional opinion. That's exactly what I did.

---

1. SIBO (Small Intestinal Bacterial Overgrowth) is a condition where excess bacteria grow in the small intestine, causing symptoms like bloating, abdominal pain, and diarrhoea. This disrupts digestion and nutrient absorption. Treatment often involves diet changes and antibiotics or antimicrobials to restore balance.

I went into the hospital with the intention of having pretty much everything done—endoscopy, colonoscopy, abdominal CAT scan, gastrointestinal tests—you name it. I was desperate, willing to give all my savings away, and ready to get better.

After a night or two in the hospital, the doctor finally came over and told me the news. Like most people who turn to "Dr. Google" in the middle of the night (which I highly recommend not doing by the way), I had convinced myself I was dealing with something more sinister—bowel cancer? A parasite? But I was ready to hear the actual diagnosis.

> "Okay, so you have Gwa-min-seong dae-jang jung-hoo-gun," the doctor explained.
>
> "Well, that was a lot longer than I was expecting," I joked, though anxiety was building.
>
> "And in English?" I asked, nervously awaiting the translation.
>
> "In English—it's irritable bowel syndrome, or IBS. You have inflammation and scarring in your large in-

> testines. We'll give you medication to aid digestion and decrease inflammation, but try to take it easy and relax. We know your symptoms, but it's hard to actually determine the cause. This can be a lifelong issue that may come and go. It's a very complex disease."

I left the hospital that day baffled and taken aback. I was handed a large shopping bag full of medication. Little did I know that I would be relying on this medication for many years to come. I would have backup pills in every pocket and wouldn't ever leave the house empty-handed. In fact, at one point, I would stop leaving the house altogether. Why leave the house when you have the protection of the toilet next to you, right?

So, if you've been diagnosed with IBS, you may be feeling confused and even a bit hopeless. You may wonder why doctors can't pinpoint the root cause or offer a simple cure. But it's crucial to understand that, while it may be frustrating, recognizing that your symptoms are part of IBS is the first step in reclaiming control over your health.

And if you can relate to this story of mine and if you're in that dark place right now like I was, please believe that you can get better. There is nothing, absolutely nothing useful down that road of self-pity and self-loathing. I know. I've been there. You can and you will get better. Believing that you can get better is very important psychologically, and I believe this will help in the long run. If you blindly accept what some doctors might say is a "lifelong" problem and you accept that as "true," then it will be. I decided not to accept that, and neither should you—which leads me on to Tip#2.

Tip #2: Believe That You Will Get Better

Managing IBS goes beyond what's on your plate—it's about understanding the powerful connection between your mind and body. The thoughts you feed your brain impact how your gut responds. By shifting your mindset to believe in the possibility of relief and reminding yourself that you are in control, you set the foundation for real change. Every day, as you explore and experiment with new approaches, know that healing is a journey, not a quick fix. Trust yourself, and remember that with patience and persistence, you have the power to improve your health. Each small step brings you closer to the peace you deserve.

Unravelling the IBS Puzzle

The challenge with IBS lies in its ever-shifting nature—it's like trying to solve a puzzle where the pieces keep changing shape. What soothes one person might leave another with no relief at all, and this unpredictability can frustrate not only those living with it but also the doctors trying to help. You've probably come across diets like low-FODMAP or elimination plans. I've tried them all, along with a mountain of medications. While they can help, there's no universal fix, because IBS stems from a tangled web of causes that often overlap, intertwine, and evolve over time.

It's not just about what you eat or how you think. There could be physical factors at play, like bacterial overgrowth, food intolerances, or a history of gut infections that leave your digestive system more sensitive. Or, it might be that your gut and brain aren't communicating smoothly, leading to an exaggerated response to stress and anxiety—almost like your body's alarm system is going off even when there's no real threat.

For some people, it might be hormone fluctuations that are throwing their system off balance. For others, it's an overly sensitive gut that reacts strongly to normal digestive processes. And let's not forget how your lifestyle choices—things like sleep, exercise, and even social interactions—can play a role in either calming your gut or setting it off. The point is, IBS is usually a mix of both internal (your mindset, stress perception, emotions) and external (food, lifestyle, physical health) factors. And that's why there's no "magic cure."

The most important thing to understand is that you'll need to experiment with different approaches—tackling both the internal and external worlds to find what works for you. No one can give you a perfect formula because it doesn't exist. But that doesn't mean you can't figure it out. It's all about creating your personalised solution.

You have to be willing to put in the work every day: figure out your unique triggers, test different strategies, and commit to making changes. And it's not just about changing what you eat or think—it's about changing how you live and approach each day. The good news? It's 100% doable. The bad news? It's going to take time, effort, and maybe a little bit of patience.

Reflection and Practical Step

Your IBS Journey

Understanding where you've come from is the first step in managing your IBS effectively. By reflecting on your experiences, you can identify patterns, triggers, and emotional responses that may have gone unnoticed. Pairing this reflection with a practical tool like a symptom diary helps you track your physical and mental state more closely. This combination can give you a clearer picture of how your IBS affects you and highlight areas where you can make adjustments to feel better. **So get a notebook and a pen, and let's get to it.**

Exercise: Reflection on Your IBS Journey

Prompt: Write about your first encounter with IBS. What were the early symptoms? How did it affect your daily life, both physically and mentally? Consider how you felt emotionally and how it impacted your relationships, work, or social life.

Practical Step: Start a symptom diary

For the next week, note down what you eat, your stress levels, and how your gut responds throughout the day. Try to include emotional responses as well. This diary can help you start identifying patterns between your food, stress, and symptoms.

Chapter 2

The Mind-Body Connection

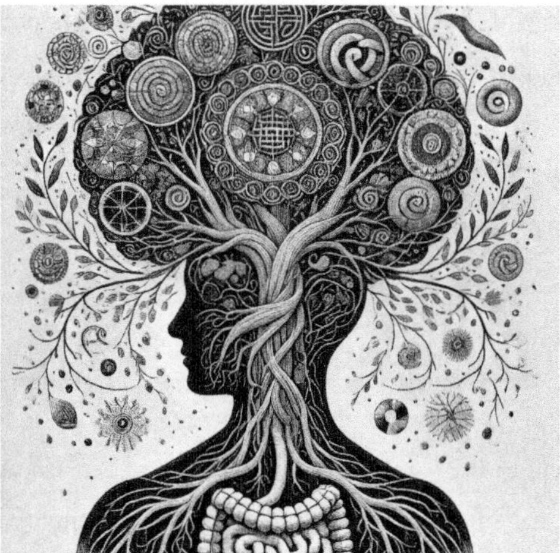

When we think about IBS, most people jump straight to food—what triggers your symptoms, what you should avoid, or what diets might help. This is all fine and well, but there's a deeper connection at play, one that goes beyond just what you put into your stomach. It's the connection between your mind and your gut—the way your thoughts, emotions, and perceptions directly impact what's happening in your digestive system.

As the British Therapist Marisa Peer[1] says, *"Your mind does what it thinks you want it to do. It listens to your words and acts on them."* This is especially relevant when it comes to managing IBS. If you constantly feed your brain with thoughts of stress and anxiety, your gut will respond accordingly. But by changing your mindset—by telling your brain that it's safe, that you're in control—you can influence how your body reacts.

The relationship between the mind and the body is powerful, and it's often underappreciated in IBS management. You might not be able to change your external circumstances, but you can control how you respond to them mentally, which has a direct impact on your gut health.

---

1. Marisa Peer is a British therapist, best-selling author, and speaker known for her work in hypnotherapy and her "Rapid Transformational Therapy" method. She focuses on helping individuals overcome limiting beliefs and achieve personal transformation through positive mental conditioning.

One of the most stressful periods of my life came when I was transitioning between jobs and countries. I was about to start a new teaching position, and the anticipation was overwhelming. My mind was doing what it loves to do, running around in circles with 'what if' scenarios: What if I wasn't good enough? What if the students didn't like me? What if I didn't get on with colleagues? My body responded immediately. The night before my first day, my stomach went into full panic mode. The cramps were unbearable, and I spent half the night in the bathroom. It wasn't until I paused, did my breathing, visualisation, grounding exercises and reminded myself that I had faced similar challenges before that my symptoms slowly began to ease. It is essential to take control of these negative automatic thoughts, page 83. By calming my mind, I was able to calm my gut. This experience highlighted the gut-brain axis (see below) for me in a way that no book or article ever could. If you're dealing with IBS, you can't just look at what's on your plate. You have to understand what's happening between your ears, too.

***

The Gut-Brain Axis - More Than Just a Gut Feeling

So this is something that sounds super technical but actually plays a huge role in how you feel every day—especially if you have IBS. The relationship between your brain and gut isn't just a passing thought—it's a full-on conversation happening 24/7. This communication is what experts call the gut-brain axis, and it's not just a metaphor for that feeling in your stomach when you're nervous. It's a literal, biochemical link between your digestive system and central nervous system, going both ways.

Think of it like a busy road, with nerves, hormones, and neurotransmitters constantly zooming back and forth between your brain and your gut. Here's why it matters: What goes on in your head affects your gut—and what's happening in your gut can change how you think and feel. It's why stress or anxiety can lead to stomach cramps or bloating, and why digestive issues can make you feel low or anxious. It's a two-way street, and it's busy.

The Role of the Vagus Nerve and Neurotransmitters

One of the key players in the gut-brain axis is the vagus nerve. Think of it as a high-speed communication motorway that runs from your brain through your body, connecting to vital organs like your heart, lungs, and, of course, your digestive system. This nerve carries messages back and forth, helping to regulate important functions like digestion, heart rate, and how your body reacts to stress.

When you're feeling relaxed, the vagus nerve signals your digestive system to get to work, making sure everything flows smoothly. But when you're stressed, it sends a different signal. It kicks your body into a "fight-or-flight" response—a state where your body is ready to react to perceived danger. This response slows down digestion and makes your gut more sensitive, leading to those all-too-familiar IBS symptoms like cramping, bloating, or needing to rush to the bathroom.

And it's not just the vagus nerve doing all the talking. Your gut and brain are constantly communicating through neurotransmitters—those tiny chemical messengers responsible for so much of what we feel. Here's something you might find surprising: about 90% of your body's serotonin—the so-called "happy hormone"—is actually produced in your gut. Serotonin doesn't just help regulate mood; it also plays a role in controlling appetite and even how you perceive pain.

What's really fascinating is how this serotonin production is linked to the health of your gut flora—the community of bacteria and other microbes living in your digestive system. When this community is balanced, everything tends to work well. But if your gut bacteria become imbalanced, it can affect your serotonin levels. This imbalance can make you feel more stressed or anxious, and it can even heighten your pain sensitivity. That's why keeping your gut healthy isn't just important for digestion; it's crucial for your emotional and mental well-being, too.

How to Support Your Vagus Nerve

The vagus nerve is a powerful ally in keeping your gut and brain in sync, and you can actively support it through simple exercises that promote relaxation and resilience. Believe it or not, you don't need fancy equipment or hours of free time—just a few simple practices can make a real difference. I'll be honest, I hadn't actually tried most of these specific exercises until I started researching for this book. But as I looked deeper, I realised that many of the activities I already do—like deep breathing and walking—must have been quietly helping to maintain my current well-being all along.

These exercises can work wonders when you're feeling stressed, helping you quickly shift out of "fight-or-flight" mode and back into "rest-and-digest." But here's the key: they're not just for moments of tension. Incorporating them into your daily routine can strengthen your vagus nerve over time, helping your body handle stress more effectively and stay calm under pressure.

Think of these practices as tools to train your nervous system for a smoother, more balanced life. Let's break down how and why they work:

Deep, Slow Breathing

Your breath is one of the simplest tools you have for calming your body and mind, and it all starts with the vagus nerve. When you breathe deeply and slowly, engaging your diaphragm, you're essentially telling your brain, "Everything's okay." This activates your parasympathetic nervous system—the one responsible for "rest-and-digest"—and helps dial down your heart rate and blood pressure. The magic lies in the exhale; making it longer than your inhale is key to creating that sense of calm.

This isn't just a relaxing exercise; it's a way to reset your system. By breathing deeply, you're giving your gut a much-needed signal to reduce sensitivity and restore smooth digestion, making it a powerful ally in managing IBS.

Techniques like diaphragmatic breathing, rhythmic breathing, and box breathing—all of which I explore in detail later in the book (see page 79)—are excellent ways to practise this. For example, the 7/11 rhythmic breathing technique, where you inhale for 7 seconds and exhale for 11 seconds, is a favourite of mine for instant calm. These methods are simple yet powerful tools to calm your body and mind, whether you're in the middle of a stressful situation or just building daily resilience.

Humming or Chanting

Ever feel the soothing effects of humming to yourself? The vibrations from humming or chanting physically stimulate the vagus nerve as it passes through the throat. This can help shift your nervous system into a calmer state while promoting feelings of connection and well-being. Singing your favourite song or repeating a mantra like "Om" can double as an enjoyable and restorative practice. It might sound a bit silly but it does actually work. Here is a video to get you started: OM chanting video (scan QR code).

Cold Exposure

Splashing your face with cold water or applying a cold compress to your neck activates the diving reflex—a natural response that slows your heart rate and redirects blood flow to vital organs. This response, mediated by the vagus nerve, helps your body step back from stress. Even short bursts of cold can "reset" your system, giving you a quick way to find calm in moments of tension.

And if you want to join the Wim Hof club, you could even start incorporating cold showers into your routine. While the idea might sound extreme, just 30 seconds of cold water at the end of your shower can have a surprising effect on both your mind and body. It activates the same vagus nerve response and leaves you feeling refreshed, calm, and even a little energised. If jumping straight into the cold isn't your thing, ease into it by alternating between warm and cool water until you feel ready to take the plunge.

Gentle Movements

Before I even knew about the vagus nerve, I started trying Tai Chi and mindful walks to manage my stress—and funnily enough, these are exactly the kinds of activities that support vagus nerve health!

Practices like yoga, tai chi, or slow, mindful walks work wonders for your vagus nerve by combining gentle movement with controlled breathing. These activities help your body shift into a calmer state, reducing stress hormones like cortisol and even lowering inflammation. Over time, they don't just make you feel more relaxed in the moment—they also build your body's ability to bounce back from everyday stress more easily.

Laughter and Connection

Here's a fun fact: genuine laughter directly stimulates the vagus nerve.[2] It reduces stress, improves mood, and even boosts your immune system—all while helping your body shift into "rest-and-digest" mode. For me, during some of the most stressful times in my life, I found myself binge-watching stand-up comedy. It was like a mini escape that gave me a good laugh and left me feeling just a little lighter afterwards.

Social bonding also plays a big role in calming your nervous system, thanks to the vagus nerve's connection to positive relationships. Whether it's catching up with a friend, sharing a joke with someone you love, or even spending time with a pet, these moments of connection aren't just good for your soul—they're good for your gut too.

Why This Matters for IBS

---

2. Zander-Schellenberg, T., Watzlawik, M., & Wilhelm, P. (2020). Does laughing have a stress-buffering effect in daily life? An intensive longitudinal study. *PLOS ONE, 15*(7), e0235851. https://doi.org/10.1371/journal.pone.0235851

Stimulating the vagus nerve isn't just about feeling calm—it's about supporting the natural balance between your gut and brain. For those managing IBS, these exercises can help ease gut motility, reduce inflammation, and even lower pain sensitivity. Over time, they contribute to a smoother digestion process and a more settled nervous system.

Adding one or two of these techniques into your daily routine doesn't need to be overwhelming. Small, consistent efforts—whether it's a few minutes of deep breathing, a mindful walk, or simply laughing more—can gradually improve how your body manages stress and responds to triggers. These simple habits can make life with IBS feel just a little more manageable.

Tip #3: Acknowledge the Mind-Gut Link

Recognise that stress, worry, and negative emotions directly affect your gut. Awareness of this connection is the first step to improving it.

The Gut Microbiota and Its Influence

By now, it's clear that the gut is far more than just a place where food is digested. It's home to a whole bustling community of bacteria, fungi, and other microbes—the gut microbiota. These tiny organisms don't just sit there quietly; they play a starring role in keeping your body functioning properly. From helping you digest food to supporting your immune system, they do a lot of heavy lifting.

A healthy, balanced gut microbiota is like having a well-tuned orchestra. When everything is in harmony, your gut can buffer stress, keep your digestion running smoothly, and even help regulate your mood. But when your gut bacteria become imbalanced—what is called dysbiosis—everything goes out of tune. This imbalance can trigger digestive issues like bloating, constipation, or diarrhoea and even lead to problems beyond your gut, like anxiety, depression, or just feeling mentally off. For those of us dealing with IBS, it's not just about the gut—it's about how everything is connected.

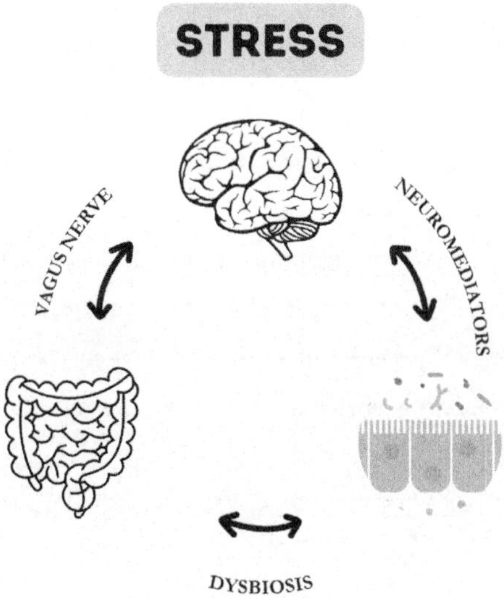

How Stress and Emotions Affect the Gut

Let's be real: when you're stressed, your body knows it. Every emotion you feel triggers a physical response, like your body's little way of echoing back what's going on in your mind. For example, when you're stressed or anxious, your brain releases cortisol, the body's main stress hormone. Now, cortisol is useful for dealing with real danger, but in our day-to-day lives, it often ends up wreaking havoc on systems like digestion.

For someone without IBS, stress might just lead to a mildly upset stomach. But for those of us with IBS, that hormonal shift can be like throwing fuel on the fire—cue the abdominal pain, bloating, urgency, or constipation.

Your gut is basically a mirror, reflecting back what's happening in your mind. Nervous about an upcoming event? Your gut will let you know. Feeling overwhelmed? Your stomach might clench up. The gut-brain connection is a two-way street, meaning that not only does your mind affect your gut, but if your gut is unhappy, it'll send signals back up to your brain, cranking up feelings of anxiety and stress. It's a feedback loop that can feel never-ending, especially when IBS flares up and you're left wondering what came first—the stress or the symptoms?

Rewiring the Gut-Brain Connection for Relief

Here's the hopeful part: just like your mind can trigger IBS symptoms, it can also help calm them down. The gut-brain axis is a two-way street, and that means you have some control over the traffic. Practices like visualisation, mindfulness, and stress management techniques can help you influence the signals that travel between your brain and gut. Essentially, you're rewiring that connection to work in your favour, creating a more relaxed, balanced digestive system.

It's incredibly empowering to realise that you're not at the mercy of your gut-brain connection. Yes, stress and anxiety might trigger symptoms, but with the right techniques, you can flip the script. By understanding how your mind and gut are linked and using strategies to manage stress and shift your thinking, you'll begin to regain control over your IBS. It's about moving from feeling helpless to feeling like you have some real tools at your disposal to manage your symptoms.

The Second Brain

When it comes to digestion, your gut actually has a mind of its own—literally. It's called the *enteric nervous system* (ENS), and it's so powerful that some people refer to it as the "second brain." Imagine a network of about 100 million nerve cells embedded right in the walls of your digestive tract, quietly managing the whole digestion process without needing any instructions from the brain in your head. This system handles essential tasks like moving food through your intestines, releasing digestive enzymes, and making sure blood flow to the gut is properly regulated. It's like having a whole control centre working behind the scenes.

Even though the ENS can function independently, it's in constant communication with your central nervous system (CNS) through the vagus nerve. This is where the gut-brain axis comes into play. It's why your emotions—like stress, anxiety, or even excitement—can trigger digestive issues. And, as many of us with IBS know all too well, when your gut is acting up, it can wreak havoc on your mental state too.

I've often thought of this gut-brain connection as a delicate dance. When things are balanced, digestion happens without much thought. But when one part is off, like when you're stressed, the whole system seems to get out of rhythm, causing chaos for your gut and your mind.

The Pain Gate Theory

When we think of pain, it's easy to assume it's just a straightforward, physical experience—like something caused by injury or irritation. But pain is far more complex than that. It's not only about what's happening in your body; it's about how your brain interprets the signals it receives. That's where the *pain gate theory* comes in.

Imagine there are literal "gates" in your spinal cord that decide whether pain signals from your body make it to your brain. These gates can either open or close. When they're open, more pain signals get through, and the pain feels sharper and more intense. When they're closed, fewer signals pass through, and the pain becomes more muted or manageable.

An interesting thing that I learned is that these gates aren't only influenced by physical factors. They're also heavily controlled by your emotional and psychological state. If you're feeling stressed, anxious, or overwhelmed, those gates swing wide open, allowing more pain signals to rush in. But when you're relaxed or distracted, the gates start to close, and the pain fades into the background.

I've definitely experienced this first-hand with IBS. There have been moments when my symptoms flared, and the stress about them just made the pain worse. But on days when I was able to calm my mind—whether through mindfulness or breathing techniques—the pain didn't feel as overwhelming. It's a powerful reminder of just how intertwined our mental and physical experiences are.

The Amygdala and the Hippocampus

There are two key players in your brain when it comes to handling stress and emotions—*the amygdala* and *the hippocampus*. Together, these regions help regulate how you feel, respond to stress, and, you guessed it, directly affect your gut.

- **The Amygdala: Fear and Anxiety**
  Think of the amygdala as your brain's personal alarm system. It processes strong emotions like fear and anxiety and triggers your fight-or-flight response—the rush of adrenaline you feel

when something stressful happens. It's a life-saver in moments of real danger, but when the amygdala stays stuck in high gear (thanks to chronic stress or anxiety), it can become a problem.

For those of us with IBS, an overactive amygdala is like having your foot permanently stuck on the gas pedal. It keeps sending distress signals to your body, which can make your gut hypersensitive to what's going on inside. This heightened alertness can amplify typical IBS symptoms like cramping, bloating, or the sudden urge to rush to the bathroom. In other words, an overworked amygdala keeps your body in a constant state of tension, making everything feel more intense.

- **The Hippocampus: Memory and Stress Regulation**
  While the amygdala sounds the alarms, the hippocampus is more like the brain's filing system. It helps regulate your emotional responses and processes memories, especially those tied to stress. You could say the hippocampus helps you "make sense" of your experiences, deciding how much of an emotional reaction they deserve.

  But when stress hangs around for too long, the hippocampus starts to lose its edge. Long-term stress can actually shrink the hippocampus[3], making it harder to regulate emotions. This is where the vicious cycle comes into play—stress shrinks the hippocampus, making it harder to manage your feelings, which in turn creates more stress. And, as we already know, stress has a direct line to our IBS symptoms[4].

Impact on the Gut

So, how do the amygdala and hippocampus end up influencing your gut? This is where the gut-brain axis steps into the spotlight once again. When your amygdala is stuck in "panic mode" and your hippocampus is struggling to process stress, your brain sends distress signals straight to your digestive system. These signals can either speed up or slow down digestion, heighten gut sensitivity, and trigger familiar IBS symptoms like pain, bloating, or irregular bowel movements.

In short: an anxious mind often equals an anxious gut. It's a two-way street—your emotional brain affects your gut health, and when your gut is upset, it sends those signals right back to your brain, making you feel even more anxious or stressed. This feedback loop can feel like a spiral, especially for people with IBS, where symptoms can start to snowball out of control.

I've been stuck in this loop more times than I'd like to admit, and I bet you have too. For instance, whenever I drink oat milk (which I love), there's a good chance it'll send me straight to the bathroom

---

3. McEwen, B. S., & Morrison, J. H. (2013). The brain on stress: Vulnerability and plasticity of the prefrontal cortex over the life course. *Neuron, 79*(1), 16–29. https://doi.org/10.1016/j.neuron.2013.06.028

with diarrhoea—not entirely sure why, but maybe it's the increase in soluble fibre. The moment my gut reacts, my anxiety flares up, and suddenly, I'm stuck in a cycle: I get anxious about the symptoms, and the anxiety makes my gut even worse. I've had days where I'm running to the bathroom all day long, even though the original trigger (the oat milk) has passed hours ago. It's a reminder of just how strong the brain-gut connection can be, and how hard it is to break free when the two are out of sync.

Managing Stress Responses

Here's the good news: just like your brain can mess things up for your gut, it can also be part of the solution. Throughout this book, I'll introduce you to practices like visualisation, mindfulness, and relaxation techniques—all of which can help retrain your brain to respond differently to stress. These practices can tone down the signals being sent to your gut, giving it a much-needed break.

By calming both your mind and your digestive system, you can break that feedback loop of anxiety and gut discomfort. The more you practise these techniques, the more you'll start to feel in control of your IBS symptoms. Stress doesn't have to rule your body's reactions anymore—with consistency, you can regain that balance and stop letting stress dictate how your gut behaves.

***

Living in the Now: Mindfulness and IBS

When I first began struggling with IBS, my mind was always somewhere else. I was constantly worried about how I'd feel tomorrow or fixated on the discomfort of yesterday's symptoms or ruminating on past events. I was stuck in a loop, worrying about what could happen next or what had gone wrong before. It wasn't until I discovered mindfulness that I realised how much time I was spending outside of the present moment.

Mindfulness is the practice of bringing your full attention to the present moment, without judgement. For someone living with IBS, this simple concept can be life-changing. By shifting your focus to what's happening *right now,* you can reduce the anxiety and stress that often trigger or worsen IBS symptoms. Instead of letting your mind wander into fearful thoughts about your body or future flare-ups, mindfulness teaches you to stay grounded in the moment. It's not just a technique to distract from anxiety—it becomes a way of life, helping you live more authentically in the present.

The beauty of mindfulness is that it doesn't ask for perfection. You don't have to eliminate all your worries or magically "fix" your gut. Instead, you focus on what's in front of you—whether it's your breath, a sensation in your body, or an activity like eating or walking. And in doing so, you begin to break the cycle of anxiety that feeds into your IBS symptoms.

This shift in mindset is powerful because, as you know, the mind and gut are closely connected through the gut-brain axis. By learning to live more in the present, you can not only calm your mind but also create a more relaxed environment for your gut, allowing your body to heal and recover without constant stress.

In the following sections, I'll take you through some simple but effective mindfulness techniques that helped me manage my IBS. These are tools that you can use anywhere, anytime, to bring yourself back to the present and soothe both your mind and your body.

The Role of Mindfulness in Managing Stress and IBS

By now, you're familiar with how closely the gut and brain are connected. We've already discussed how stress can intensify IBS symptoms, but the real challenge is learning how to break that cycle in the moment. This is where mindfulness can play a powerful role.

Mindfulness is all about being fully present—right here, right now. It's about paying attention to the moment without letting your thoughts and emotions spiral. (Later on, you will learn grounding techniques, which are a part of a mindfulness practice). When you feel your IBS symptoms creeping in, the natural reaction is panic: What if this gets worse? What if I can't leave the house? These thoughts lead to stress, and the stress only worsens the symptoms. It's a vicious loop, one I know all too well.

The practice of mindfulness teaches us to observe what's happening in our body and mind without getting swept away by it. By bringing your attention to the present moment and focusing on your breath or sensations, you can stop the stress response before it takes over. You create space between the feeling of anxiety and your reaction to it.

Eckhart Tolle[5] captures this beautifully when he says, *"Realise deeply that the present moment is all you have. Make the NOW the primary focus of your life."* When you truly live in the present, you can avoid the mental spiralling that so often aggravates IBS symptoms.

Instead of letting your thoughts run wild, mindfulness lets you ground yourself in what's actually happening—not what you fear might happen. By practising mindfulness regularly, you can begin to ease that mind-gut tension and take the power back from your symptoms.

In the next section, we'll dive into some practical mindfulness exercises that I've found especially useful for managing IBS-related stress.

Mindfulness in Action: Simple Practices for IBS Relief

Mindfulness is often associated with meditation, but it's much more than that. It's about cultivating awareness in your daily life, and for

---

5. Eckhart Tolle is a spiritual teacher and author, best known for his books *The Power of Now* and *A New Earth*. His teachings focus on mindfulness, presence, and the transformative power of living in the present moment to overcome negative thought patterns and find inner peace.

those of us with IBS, it can be a lifeline when symptoms start to flare. The key is to integrate mindfulness into everyday activities so that it becomes a natural response to stress, rather than an afterthought.

Here are a few practical techniques I've found helpful

1. **Mindful Breathing**
   One of the simplest and most effective mindfulness practices is mindful breathing. When you feel stress or anxiety building up, take a few moments to focus solely on your breath. Slowly inhale through your nose for a count of four, hold your breath for four, and exhale through your mouth for a count of four. This method, known as box breathing, can quickly calm your body and mind. You can also try 7/11 breathing, where you inhale through your nose for seven counts and exhale out your mouth for eleven. (More on that in chapter 3) The key is to be fully present with each breath, completely focused on the rhythm. By doing so, you calm your nervous system and ease the gut-brain tension that often triggers IBS symptoms. Afterwards, you can also simply just focus on your breath without trying to follow any specific rhythm. Just watch your breath, notice how your body doesn't need you to consciously think about it. I find this to be especially helpful with staying in the present.

2. **Body Scanning**
   This technique helps you tune in to what's happening in your body without judgement. Starting from the top of your head, mentally scan down through each part of your

body, noticing where you might be holding tension. When you reach your stomach, pay particular attention to how it feels. Instead of fighting the discomfort, acknowledge it. Just bringing awareness to the sensations without resistance can help reduce the emotional intensity tied to IBS symptoms. There are some helpful videos on page 179 and page 184.

3. **Mindful Eating**

   IBS often turns mealtimes into a source of anxiety. But mindful eating can help you reconnect with your body's natural hunger and fullness cues. Before you eat, take a moment to appreciate the food in front of you. Eat slowly, savouring each bite, and focus on the flavours, textures, and smells. Chew thoroughly and pause between bites to notice how your stomach feels. This practice can reduce overeating, minimise stress around food, and give your digestive system time to properly process each meal. (I explore this in more depth on page 338.)

4. **Mindfulness During Daily Activities**

   You don't need to set aside large chunks of time to practise mindfulness. One of the most transformative changes I made was learning to be mindful during specific activities—things as simple as brushing my teeth, taking a shower, or having dinner. These everyday tasks became opportunities to ground myself in the present, instead of letting my mind race ahead to worries or symptoms. By staying mindful in these moments, I created a sense of calm that carried over into the rest of my day.

"The primary cause of unhappiness is never the situation but your thoughts about it."

Eckhart Tolle

Applying mindfulness to routine activities allows you to take control of your thoughts, reducing the anxiety that often fuels IBS symptoms. By incorporating these small, mindful actions into your daily life, you can build resilience to stress and help reduce the impact of IBS on your physical and emotional well-being.

Breaking the Illusion of Time: Living in the Now

One of the most liberating realisations I've ever had is that our entire experience exists in the present moment—there's no past or future that we can directly access. The present moment is the only time we truly have control over. As Lao Tzu[6] says, "*If you are depressed, you*

---

6. Lao Tzu was an ancient Chinese philosopher and the founder of Daoism, best known for authoring the *Tao Te Ching*. His teachings emphasise living in harmony with the Dao (or "the Way"), embracing simplicity, humility, and the principle of *wu wei*—effortless action or non-striving—allowing life to unfold naturally.

are living in the past. If you are anxious, you are living in the future. If you are at peace, you are living in the present".[7] This is a simple yet profound truth, and when it comes to managing IBS, understanding and embracing it can help alleviate a lot of the anxiety and stress we create around our symptoms.

We tend to think of time as this linear thing—a never-ending stretch between the past, present, and future. But in reality, as we experience it, the past and future are just concepts. They don't exist except in our minds. It's like wearing orange-tinted glasses when skiing. When you put them on, the snow appears orange. You forget you're looking through a filter, and it feels as if the world is truly that colour. Similarly, we experience time through the filter of our minds, but that doesn't mean it exists the way we think it does.

This might sound abstract, but think about it: when you worry about the future, what's actually happening? You're creating a stressful experience in the present moment by imagining something that hasn't happened yet. The same goes for ruminating on the past—your

---

7. While Lao Tzu's quote provides a timeless perspective on the importance of living in the present, it's important to recognize that depression is sometimes rooted in an imbalance in brain chemistry or other biological factors. This quote, which originates from ancient wisdom, may not fully capture the complexity of modern mental health conditions. Nonetheless, its overarching message about the value of presence and mindfulness holds significant practical wisdom for many people.

thoughts are happening *now*, and they're affecting how you feel in the present. But the past isn't a place you can revisit. It's only a memory in your mind, and the future is just a projection.

Living mindfully helps you break free from the anxiety tied to these imagined scenarios. By focusing on what's happening *right now*, you reduce the power that stress about the future or regret about the past has over you. This is especially important for those of us with IBS, where stress is a key trigger. When you train your mind to stay in the present, you stop feeding that vicious cycle of anxiety and symptoms.

Long-Term Benefits of Mindfulness for IBS

When I first started practising mindfulness, it wasn't easy, and I wasn't expecting miracles. I started small and with specific activities one by one, like brushing my teeth, eating, showering, and going for walks. But over time, I began to notice subtle shifts. It wasn't that the stress or the IBS completely disappeared overnight—far from it. But the way I *handled* stress began to change. I began to react less to stress, noticing my body didn't immediately respond with gut-wrenching discomfort. The more I practised staying present, the less I let my mind spiral into the endless loop of "what ifs" and "why me?"

Gradually, I felt calmer, more in control, and less at the mercy of my symptoms. My gut didn't seem to react so violently every time I faced stress. It wasn't just that mindfulness helped in the moment—it was that it began to change how I responded to stress on a day-to-day

Mindset is everything when it comes to managing IBS. So if you're constantly telling yourself that you'll never get better, your body will respond to that negativity. On the other hand, if you believe that you can heal and improve, you're setting the foundation for real change. It doesn't mean that symptoms will vanish overnight, but it shifts how you approach your condition.

There was a point in my journey where I felt utterly defeated. My symptoms were worse than ever, and I was convinced that this was how my life would always be—constantly revolving around bathroom breaks, dietary restrictions, and stress. It wasn't until I started challenging that belief, though, that things began to change. I remember the moment clearly: I was sitting at home after a particularly rough day at work, and I just thought, 'I can't keep living like this.' Something clicked, and I decided to take responsibility for my health. I focused on the small victories—days where my symptoms were mild, or when I managed to stay calm under pressure. I learned new techniques for managing my negative mind and to relax. Gradually, my mindset shifted from defeat to hope. This belief, I realised, was the foundation for real progress.

Believing that you can get better doesn't mean ignoring the tough days or pretending everything is perfect. It means acknowledging your challenges while staying open to the possibility of improvement. Your mindset is a key tool in breaking the cycle of stress and symptoms, and it all starts with believing in your ability to heal.

Once I realised that my mindset was essential, I understood that I couldn't wait around for some external fix. I couldn't just hope that the next pill or diet would magically solve all my problems. I had to take responsibility for my own health, and actively make the necessary changes in my life. That's when real progress began. And now it's your turn to do the same.

Taking Responsibility: The Hard Part

Mindset is the foundation, but mindset alone won't carry you. Believing you can heal is the starting point, but it's the actions you take that will bring real progress. And here's where things get tough. It's easy to say, "I'll try anything." It's easy to hope for change. But actually following through? That's a whole different story.

In my experience, this is the part where most people (myself included) stumble. I've met many others with IBS who *want* to feel better but struggle to take responsibility and take meaningful action. Let me be completely honest: IBS is frustrating, and it's easy to fall into a mindset of resentment. Why should you have to give up your favourite foods? Why should you be the one who has to make all these changes when it feels like everyone else around you is eating and living without a second thought? It's just not fair.

I used to think this way, too. I resented the fact that I had to make sacrifices. I hated that beer, coffee, and pastries—things I loved—triggered my symptoms. I hated that my friends could live exactly how they wanted without having to worry about finding the nearest toilet. But here's the thing: if you want to get better, you're going to have to give some things up, at least in the beginning. I'm not going to sugarcoat it: this part sucks. Letting go of habits and foods you love is hard, especially when it feels like everyone else around you can live without a second thought. But how badly do you want to feel better?

To move forward, you need to let go of resentment and shift your focus from 'Why me?' to 'What can I do?'

Moving Beyond the "Why Me?" Mentality

So, when faced with gut issues that demand lifestyle changes, it's natural to think, "Why me? Why should I have to change everything—what I eat, my routines, my entire life?" If you feel this way, know that you're not alone. Many of us with chronic gut problems have been there, wondering why our bodies seem to need extra care and attention. But staying in this mindset can hold you back from real healing.

The first step is acceptance. Acknowledge your current reality: the truth is that your body isn't functioning optimally right now and needs support to recover. Accepting this is not about giving up—it's about giving yourself permission to heal. Embrace the idea that good health often requires time, effort, and, yes, a bit of sacrifice. Think of it as an investment in your long-term well-being, one that will pay off with resilience, comfort, and freedom from constant worry.

Reframe the "Why Me?"

Instead of dwelling on why this is happening, try asking yourself, "How can I respond to this in a way that helps me feel better?" Shifting from a place of frustration to a place of empowerment can turn this journey into one of growth and resilience. It's not easy, but it's worth it.

Focus on One Step at a Time

When you look at everything you might need to do, it can feel overwhelming. I remember, as a kid, I was scared of heights. So, my dad naturally would take me on hikes up mountains like Helvellyn and Scafell Pike! At the start, I'd look at the peak and think it was too high, too far, and would take too long to reach. It seemed impossible. But he'd remind me to focus on just putting one foot in front of the other—and, if possible, to enjoy the process along the way. The more I focused on each small step, rather than the entire climb, the easier the journey became. And before I knew it, I'd be at the top.

So, approach your healing journey the same way. Each small step—whether it's applying the advice and techniques from this book, like preparing a gut-friendly meal, practising stress management, or skipping that morning coffee—adds up. It may feel like you're barely making progress, but those steps accumulate. Focus on one change, one day at a time, and trust that, eventually, you'll look back and realise just how far you've come.

Choose Your Path

Imagine yourself standing at a crossroads. One path involves staying where you are, with familiar habits and routines that may keep your symptoms steady or worsening—like continuing to eat trigger foods, ignoring stress management, or hoping for change without taking action. The other path is one of change—adopting new habits and routines to support your health. This choice is yours to make. It's okay if the journey feels tough, but know that you have the power to choose a healthier, more fulfilling path.

Be Kind to Yourself

I think this is a really important point. Remember not to be hard on yourself for feeling frustrated or resistant. Chronic health challenges are tough. Practice self-compassion, understanding that these struggles don't define you. You're on a journey, and it's okay to go at your own pace.

Embrace the Process, Not Just the Destination

This journey isn't just about "fixing" your body; it's about building a life that supports you in feeling your best. Every time you make a positive choice for yourself—whether it's choosing a gut-friendly meal or taking a moment to breathe through stress—you're building a healthier future. The goal isn't perfection but progress. Remember, every step you take is part of your healing, and each one is worth celebrating.

Let's be honest: it's not easy to give up habits and foods you love. But ask yourself, how badly do you want to feel better? Are you willing to give up coffee, alcohol, or that weekly takeaway if it means your stomach can finally calm down? How willing are you to embrace these changes if they could lead to a real improvement in your quality of life?

This journey requires honesty and commitment. Take a moment to reflect on what you truly want. How much are you prepared to invest in feeling better—not just for today, but for the long term? The choice is yours. Each step you take—no matter how small—is a step toward the possibility of a healthier, more comfortable life.

***

Managing Worry: Hypothetical vs. Practical Worry

Worry is one of the biggest triggers for IBS flare-ups. But not all worries are the same, and separating them can make a huge difference in how you cope. One technique that has helped me immensely is categorising worries into two types: **hypothetical worries** (the "what ifs") and **practical worries** (the actionable kind).

Hypothetical vs. Practical Worries

- **Hypothetical Worries**: These are the "what if" worries—like "What if I have a flare-up during the meeting?" or "What if I embarrass myself?" Often irrational and beyond our control, these worries spiral without resolution.
- **Practical Worries**: These are specific problems that can be solved, such as "I have a meeting tomorrow, so I'll prepare a safe meal and bring my medication just in case." These worries allow proactive steps.

Tip #4: Separate Hypothetical and Practical Worries

Start a worry diary to separate hypothetical and practical worries. Write down what you're worrying about, then ask yourself, "Is this something I can control right now?" If it's practical, take action. If it's hypothetical, try to let it go.

The Worry Tree

A practical method for managing your worries is to visualise a "worry tree." This tool guides you to decide what to do with a concern. Please see the image on the next page:

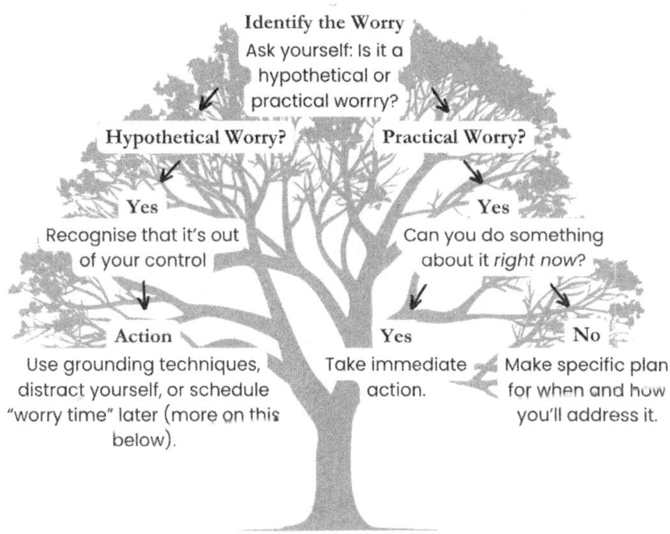

Worry Time: The Art of Controlled Worrying

If you're like I was (and most people dealing with IBS), worries have a way of creeping up all day long, like those unsolicited emails that keep popping into your inbox. But here's the deal: *you get to decide when to open them*. That's where "Worry Time" comes in—a technique that gives your worries a VIP pass to your attention, but only when *you* say so.

What Is Worry Time, Anyway?

It's like putting your worries in a little box with a time-lock. You dedicate a specific 20-minute window each day to let it all out. Think of it as a "worry free-for-all." During this time, it's an anything-goes session where you give your mind the space to do all the worrying it craves. After that, worry time is up, and you lock that box away until tomorrow.

Sounds simple, right? That's because it is. By giving your worries a defined space to roam free, they won't sneak up on you throughout the day, demanding attention at the most inconvenient times (like right before bed, when you're in the shower, or mid-coffee sip).

How to Nail Down Your Worry Time Routine

1. **Pick Your "Worry Window."** Choose a set 20-minute slot during the day—something consistent works best (after work is always best for me). But don't make it right before bed. You don't want to turn your pillow into a "Worry Headquarters."

2. **Jot Down Those Worries.** Throughout the day, when a worry pops up, scribble it down (I just write it in a note on my phone) and tell yourself, "I'll deal with this later."

3. **Unleash the Worries (But Only in That Window).** When your scheduled time arrives, go through your list. Let yourself stew, stress, and fret about everything on there—it's a judgement-free zone. If anything feels resolved or, in hindsight, totally ridiculous, cross it off the list. And once those 20 minutes are up, worry time is officially *closed*.

4. **Move On to Something You Love.** Once the timer goes off, it's time to shake it off and do something that makes you happy. Walk it out, brew a tea, play your favourite song—whatever helps you press the reset button. It's essential that you do something relaxing and enjoyable straight after!

Top Tips to Keep You on Track

- **Stick to Worrying**

  It might feel a bit strange to focus exclusively on worrying, but hey, you set this time aside for it—use it! If your mind starts drifting off into "non-worry" territory (lucky you!), just gently steer it back to the list.

- **Keep a Worry Diary**

  Write those worries down throughout the day, like they're mental "notes to self." Like I said, using a phone was easier for me but others prefer to actually write it down. Remember, the more you practise catching and postponing them, the more in control you'll feel.

- **Set a Timer and Stick to It**

  Like a Netflix binge, worry time can be all-consuming. Keep it to 20 minutes max! This way, you don't let those worries sprawl into an hours-long ordeal.

- **Don't Sweat Consistency**

  If your schedule is a bit all over the place, aim for the same time after a regular daily activity, like lunch or after a workout. The routine will help your brain learn, "Okay, this is when we worry, and this is when we don't."

Remember: Practice Makes Progress

It might feel awkward at first—setting time aside just to worry. It did take me a while to make it into a routine. But over time, you'll notice something magical happening: your brain will get used to "saving it for later." Your worries won't have the same hold over your day because they know they'll get their turn. This activity really does help and I hope you start it from today! Don't wait!

Tip #5: Set Worry Time

Dedicate 20 minutes each day to focus on worries, then set them aside. This practice helps prevent worry from creeping into your day and affecting your gut.

Ruminating

If you're anything like me, you might find yourself going over and over situations in the past. These could be situations from the day, last week, a month ago, or even years ago! I used to find myself going over things that happened even 20 years ago. This is called rumination—the repetitive and passive thinking about negative feelings, problems, or distress.

For rumination about the past, it's very simple. Allow yourself only 2 minutes to ruminate using a timer. Use this time to let it all out, replay the situation, and feel whatever you need to feel. But afterwards, take a deep breath and ask yourself these three questions:

- **Did thinking about the past help me in any way now?**
  This question helps you identify if your rumination is bringing any positive outcomes or simply keeping you stuck. Often, it highlights that the thinking process is not as useful as it seems.

- **What did I learn from this situation that could be applied to the present?**
  By seeking a lesson or insight, you can transform rumination into a more constructive reflection. This makes your thoughts actionable and allows you to focus on how to move forward.

- **If I could let go of these thoughts, what would I gain or be free to do?**
  Visualising the benefits of letting go can motivate you to

release these thoughts. It focuses on the possibilities and opportunities that come with moving beyond the past.

The best way I have found to make use of these questions is to write them down in Notes on my phone so I'm ready to have them at hand when I start ruminating and I set myself a timer. Alternatively, you could write them down on a piece of paper in case you are in the 5% of people who don't own a phone!

So, once you've answered these questions, it's time to take action. Here's are some tips:

Take Action or Make a Plan

If any of the questions revealed something actionable—like a lesson learned or a step you can take—do it. Whether it's making a decision, reaching out to someone, or writing down what you learned for future reference, take a proactive approach. It's easy to tell yourself you'll act later, but the truth is that small, quick actions are often the most effective in breaking the rumination cycle.

For a while, I thought I had said something wrong to a colleague, and I was convinced she was avoiding me or acting strangely around me. I kept ruminating, going over the situation in my head. Eventually, I realised I had two options: either move on and ignore it, or address it directly with her. But I couldn't just stay in this loop. Even if she chose to lie and say everything was fine when it might not have been, I knew I had done my part by bringing it up.

So, I decided to address it. We sat down, had a good talk about what had been bothering me, and cleared the air. It turned out there was in fact a small issue, but we were able to move on successfully. Afterwards, we worked even better together, and making decisions like this has greatly improved my work life.

The experience taught me that it's no good just deciding to act; you have to follow through, even if it feels uncomfortable. By addressing the situation, I broke the rumination cycle, and our working relationship improved as a result. Taking action—whether it's clarifying something with someone or writing down your thoughts—puts you back in control and prevents rumination from taking over.

Refocus on the Present

Bring your awareness back to the present moment. Use the grounding exercises I discuss in Chapter 3, page 73 (the 5-4-3-2-1 method). Basically, you focus on your senses—what you can see, hear, touch, taste, and smell—to reconnect with what's happening right now. This helps to centre you and pull your attention away from those repetitive thoughts. Mindful breathing and body scanning can also be helpful.

Distract Yourself with a Positive Activity

Engage in something enjoyable or meaningful to break the cycle of rumination. Go for a walk, listen to your favourite music, or start a hobby that requires your full attention. The key is to engage your mind and body in something uplifting.

Practise Self-Compassion

Recognise that everyone ruminates from time to time. Be kind to yourself, acknowledge that it's okay to make mistakes or feel regret, and remind yourself that growth often comes from learning to let go.

Use Visualisation Techniques

Picture yourself literally letting go of the thought. Imagine placing it on a leaf that floats away down a stream or on a balloon that drifts off into the sky. This imagery can help you mentally release those lingering worries. (More on visualisation on page 93)

The point of these exercises is to give yourself a structured way to process your thoughts and then move on. It might feel strange at first, but with practice, it becomes easier to let go of the past and focus on living in the present. Since I tend to ruminate a lot, I like to keep the questions and these extra techniques in a note on my phone and I have used them every day for a long time until the automatic worries slowly started to disappear. But I really recommend putting it all on your phone, otherwise you'll end up like I was going "What was the second question again?" and then you give up and continue to ruminate throughout the day without ever getting over it. You'll likely find that as you get better at identifying and addressing rumination, your mental clarity and peace of mind will greatly improve.

App Recommendation

If you'd like to use a digital tool to manage your worries, try the **WorryTree app**. It provides a simple, structured approach to managing anxiety by guiding users through identifying and addressing their worries. It helps break down concerns into manageable steps, allowing you to decide whether to take action or let go of hypothetical worries. It's easy-to-use and has daily reminders. I personally think it's really good to use at the start to make you more consistent with identifying and then managing your worries.

However, the app does have a fixed structure and might feel a bit repetitive for some users, and it lacks in-depth resources about anxiety or cognitive behavioural therapy (CBT) techniques. I used it at the start and when I got into the swing of things I was able to use notes and I also have a notebook at hand as well. They do offer a free trial for a week though, so you can see if it works for you before committing to a monthly or yearly plan. It's an accessible tool for those seeking a straightforward way to manage worries! Just a thought.

The Vicious Cycle: Breaking the Chain

I am certain you already know this by now but IBS often creates a vicious cycle that seems impossible to escape:

1. You worry about your IBS causing problems.

2. Anxiety and nervousness build quickly.

3. Symptoms occur.

4. Foods or situations trigger or increase those symptoms.

5. The worry increases, and the cycle continues.

This cycle can trap you. It certainly trapped me. I was constantly on edge, wondering if my IBS would act up at the worst possible moment. And guess what? That very anxiety and anticipation made the symptoms even worse. It was a self-fulfilling prophecy.

The key to breaking the cycle is to address both sides: your mindset and your actions. You need to reduce stress, manage your thoughts, and calm your body. This might sound overwhelming at first, but once you start to understand how it works, it becomes more manageable.

***

The 5 Areas Model

IBS isn't just about isolated symptoms—it's a complex interplay between different aspects of your life. That's where the **5 Areas Model** comes in. This model provides a way to break down and understand how your **thoughts, emotions, physical sensations, behaviours,** and **life situations** all link together to create the cycle of IBS. It's like a web: each area impacts the others, sometimes in obvious ways, sometimes in subtler ones.

The beauty of the 5 Areas Model is that it allows you to see how a single thought or life event can set off a chain reaction throughout your entire experience, affecting your emotions, physical sensations, and even your behaviours. For example, a stressful situation at work can trigger anxious thoughts, which lead to certain emotions, physical symptoms like stomach cramps, and behaviours such as avoiding certain foods or situations. By understanding these connections, you're better equipped to identify where you can break the cycle and find relief.

The goal is to recognise the patterns and interactions in your own life. When you see how these five areas interact, you can begin to make small changes in one area that ripple out to the others—whether it's shifting your perspective on a challenging situation, finding ways to manage stress, or changing your behaviour to reduce physical symptoms. This model doesn't just help you understand the "why" of your IBS; it helps you find practical pathways to manage it effectively.

Below is a visual representation:

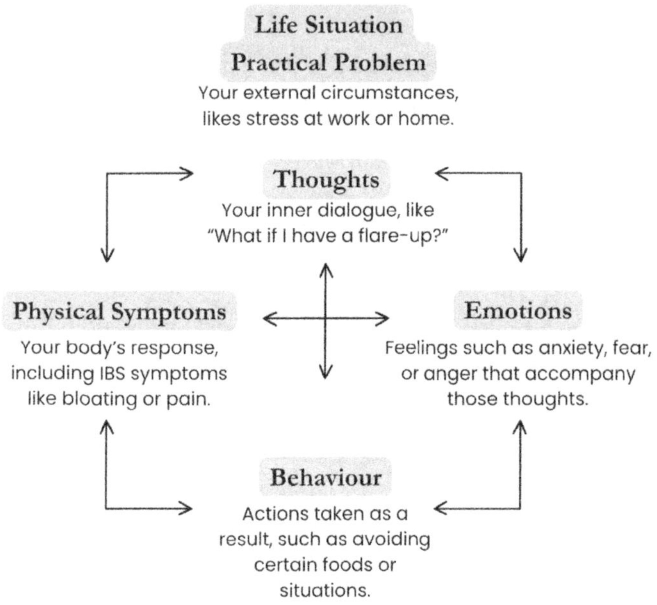

You're in Control

At the end of the day, you're in control of your health journey. Yes, IBS can feel like it's taking over your life, but the truth is, you have more power than you think. You can make choices that will improve your symptoms. You can manage stress in ways that calm your gut.

You can change how you eat, sleep, and live to create a more peaceful and symptom-free life.

But remember: it starts with belief. If you don't believe you can get better, you won't. The mind is incredibly powerful—do not underestimate it.

Reflection and Practical Step

Exploring the Mind-Body Connection

Now that you've explored the powerful connection between your mind and gut, it's time to apply these insights to your personal experience. Take a moment to reflect on how your thoughts, emotions, and stress levels impact your IBS. This personal awareness can reveal patterns and triggers unique to you. By introducing simple yet powerful practices—like mindfulness, setting aside 'Worry Time,' and the 2-minute rumination rule—you'll gain practical tools to manage anxiety and stress with confidence, calming both mind and body for a smoother path forward.

Exercise: Reflection on Stress Triggers

> **Prompt:** Reflect on a time when you felt your IBS symptoms were triggered by stress or emotional turmoil. How did your body respond, and what was the situation that caused it? Consider the physical symptoms, the emotions you were experiencing, and how they affected your gut.

Practical Step: Practise Worry Time and the 2-Minute Rumination Rule.

- **Worry Time:** Set aside 20 minutes each day as your designated worry window. Throughout the day, jot down any stressful or anxious thoughts, but save them for this specific time. When the time comes, review your list, allow yourself to fully process those worries, then put them aside until the next session.
- **2-Minute Rumination Rule:** If you find yourself ruminating about a past event, allow yourself only 2 minutes to dwell on it. Use a timer, then ask yourself: Did thinking about this help me? What did I learn from it? And, what can I gain by letting it go?

Tracking your progress with these practices will help you reduce the impact of stress on your IBS and gain control over your thought patterns.

Chapter 3

Breaking the Vicious Cycle

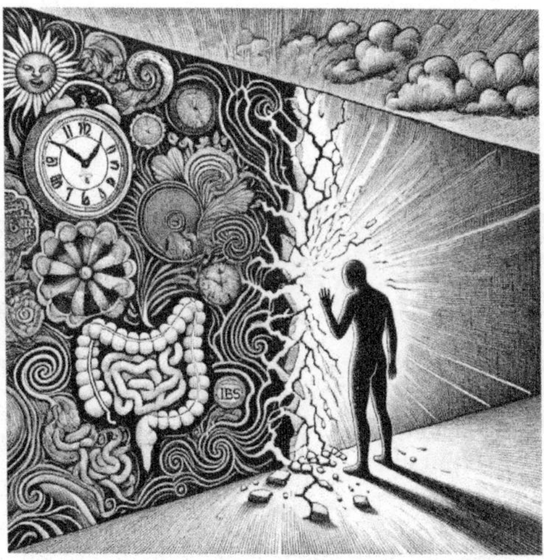

When you feel those familiar pangs of anxiety, it's like standing at the edge of a cliff. The cycle seems relentless. But you're not alone—I've been on that cliff, too, convinced I might fall at any moment. And guess what? I learned how to step back, breathe, and find my balance. It starts with small shifts. In this chapter, I will talk about different breathing techniques, along with other strategies to help you take control of your anxiety before it spirals. From shifting your mindset to finding ways to ground yourself in the present, these tools can work together to help you break the cycle of stress. Remember that practice makes progress. When you try these exercises out, every time you breathe out, imagine letting go of just a bit of that anxiety. You've got this.

As Marisa Peer wisely said, *"The most important words you will ever hear are the words you say to yourself."* This couldn't be more relevant when it comes to managing IBS. Your inner dialogue plays a huge role in determining how your body reacts to stress and anxiety, which, in turn, affects your IBS symptoms. When negative thoughts dominate your mind, they feed into the vicious cycle of anxiety and symptoms. But when you shift your self-talk toward positivity, your body can start to follow suit.

One of the most powerful tools you have in managing IBS doesn't come from a doctor or a diet—it comes from your own mind. It might sound cliché, but science is starting to back it up: what you expect can truly shape your physical reality. In his book *The Expectation Effect*, David Robson explores how our thoughts and expectations directly influence how we feel, both mentally and physically. This is especially relevant when it comes to chronic conditions like IBS, where your mindset plays an active role in managing symptoms.

For instance, Robson points out how our expectations alone can impact physical health. If we expect to feel pain, discomfort, or anxiety, those very symptoms are often amplified, as if our brain is primed for them. This is known as the "nocebo effect," the counterpart to the placebo effect, where negative expectations can worsen symptoms just as positive expectations can improve them. When you believe that you won't get better, that your symptoms will only get worse, your brain essentially takes that as instruction. It anticipates pain, discomfort, and stress, and as a result, your body responds accordingly. This can create a self-fulfilling prophecy, where the expectation of anxiety or symptoms unintentionally reinforces those very experiences. Your gut, which is already hypersensitive due to IBS, becomes even more reactive. This is where the gut-brain axis comes into play—your thoughts and perceptions are closely tied to what happens in your digestive system.

On the flip side, if you start to expect improvement, research shows that this can actually have a physiological effect on your body. It's not just about positive thinking—it's about setting a realistic expectation that things can and will get better with the right tools and strategies. When you expect to feel calmer or less bloated, your body starts to align with those beliefs, helping to break the vicious cycle of anxiety and gut issues.

If you've lived with IBS for any length of time, you know all too well the vicious cycle that comes with it: symptoms flare up, you get anxious about the symptoms, and that anxiety just makes everything worse. It's a cruel loop—anxiety causes symptoms, symptoms cause more anxiety, and on it goes. It's like a digestive merry-go-round, except nobody's having any fun, and you're definitely not lining up to go again!

For years, I was caught in this cycle, and breaking free felt almost impossible. But it's not. You can break the cycle, and you can regain control of your life.

When that first wave of anxiety hits, or when you feel the first twinge in your stomach, you have the opportunity to break the cycle. This is where techniques like rhythmic breathing (page 80) and visualisation (page 93) come into play. The key is to act quickly before your anxiety spirals and your symptoms worsen.

There was one afternoon where I found myself caught in a vicious loop. I was invited to a large social gathering, and the thought of socialising immediately triggered my anxiety. I'm not sure why, but my mind went straight to, 'What if I need to use the bathroom urgently? What if there's no place to go?' As I felt my stomach start to twist, I knew I had to act fast. I stopped what I was doing and practised my 7/11 breathing for three minutes. At first, my thoughts kept pulling me back to my worries, but I stayed focused. Slowly, I could feel the tension in my gut easing and my heart rate slowing down. By the time I finished, I felt more in control. The anxiety seems to feed off of those negative automatic thoughts, so it's very important to reassure yourself. Sure, It wasn't perfect for me, but it was enough for me to go to the party and enjoy myself.

This is why it's so important to have tools like rhythmic breathing, visualisation, grounding, and especially being able to notice, challenge and reframe your thoughts. So that you are ready when you feel anxiety building. Practising these techniques below will help break the cycle and give you back control over your symptoms before they take over.

But to understand how these techniques work, we first need to break down the cycle itself. By understanding the steps of the anxiety-symptom loop, you'll see where you can intervene and use the tools effectively.

Understanding the Cycle

Here's a closer look:

1. **The Initial Trigger**: Maybe it's a stressful meeting at work, a social event, or even just a lingering worry in the back of your mind. Something sparks anxiety, and if you're like me, your gut reacts almost instantly.

2. **Physical Symptoms Begin**: A cramp, bloating, or that awful urgency to find a bathroom. Whatever it is, your body kicks into IBS mode. And what's the first thing that happens when you start to feel those symptoms? You get even more anxious.

3. **Anxiety Amplifies Symptoms**: Now, instead of calming down, your body goes into overdrive. You start worrying about the symptoms—"Will I make it to a bathroom? Will

I embarrass myself? Am I going to have to leave?" The more you think about it, the worse the symptoms get.

4. **The Cycle Continues**: And here's the thing—your body doesn't know how to get off this ride. The anxiety makes your gut react, and your gut reacting makes your anxiety worse. So the symptoms stay, or they get worse, and you find yourself in a state of constant stress and discomfort.

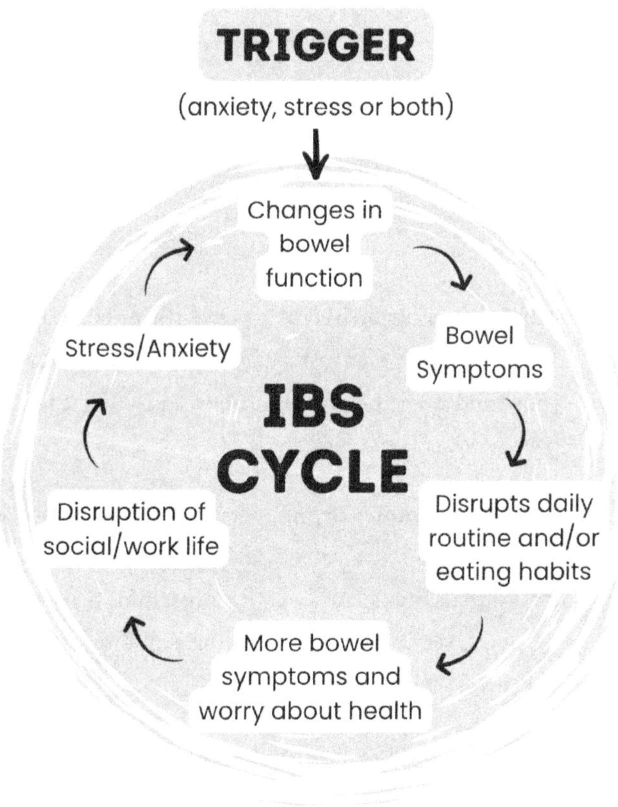

It's a never-ending loop... unless you decide to break it.

Tip #6: Break the Cycle Before It Breaks You

The key to breaking this vicious cycle is in the moments when it begins—when that first wave of anxiety hits, or when you feel the first twinge in your stomach. This is where you can take control, and it starts with rewiring how you respond, both physically and mentally.

Relaxation Exercises: Breathing

A few years ago, I had to give a speech to a few hundred people. Naturally, I was nervous, so a friend came up to me and said, "Just take a few deep breaths and try to relax!" Now, at that moment, I sarcastically thought to myself, *Oh, fantastic! Deep breaths, you say? If only someone had told me that before!* It felt as useful as someone saying, "Mind the step!" after you've already tripped.

I remember vividly a time when I was stuck in traffic in a taxi—one of my mind's favourite places to spiral into anxiety. I was, of course, far away from any bathroom, and I could feel my stomach starting to churn. Panic set in as my body prepared for the worst. In that moment, I decided to practise the 7/11 breathing technique (along with some visualisation I'd practised beforehand). At first, I was sceptical—how could something so simple help? But as I focused on my breath, counting seven seconds in and eleven seconds out, the tightness in my stomach began to release. The urgency that had felt overwhelming started to fade, and by the time I arrived, I didn't even need to stop. That was a turning point for me—realising I had more control over my symptoms than I thought.

But the truth is, there **is** something to this whole "deep breathing" thing. It's scientifically proven that certain breathing patterns can help calm the nervous system and reduce anxiety. The idea isn't just to take a few quick gasps of air, but to actually focus on your breathing rhythm in a controlled way and do it for at least 3-5 minutes at the start.

In fact, when I had to give a wedding speech not long after that, I decided to give these breathing techniques a real try. Thankfully, the speech went smoothly—though I have to admit, I was also armed with some anti-diarrhoea tablets, just in case!

Rhythmic Breathing

We breathe every day without thinking about it. But breathing isn't just about getting oxygen into your body—it's one of the most powerful ways to influence your nervous system. When you're stressed, anxious, or overwhelmed, your breathing often becomes shallow and rapid, triggering your body's "fight or flight" response. But here's where rhythmic breathing comes in: by intentionally slowing down and controlling your breath, you can actively switch on your "rest and digest" system—the parasympathetic nervous system—which helps to calm your mind and relax your body.

The concept of rhythmic breathing is simple, but it can be incredibly effective.

Here's how you do it:

1. **Breathe with a fixed ratio of 'in' to 'out'**. It doesn't matter what the ratio is as long as it's fixed. However, breathing with a longer out-breath is generally better for activating the parasympathetic nervous system. Try 4 seconds in and 6 seconds out, or 6 in and 8 out. The key is consistency.

2. **Keep your breathing smooth and even**. Avoid erratic breaths or quick inhalations. Aim for a calm, steady rhythm.

3. **Focus your attention on your chest**. This may seem odd, but focusing on the chest area instead of your abdomen helps you avoid overthinking. This approach is especially effective because your heart generates more electrical power than any other part of your body. When you focus here, you connect with positive emotions and can quiet the chatter in your head.

7/11 Breathing: My favourite rhythmic breathing ratio

One of the most effective rhythmic breathing ratios I've found is **7/11 breathing**. It's the same as above but here's how it works:

- Inhale through your nose for 7 seconds.
- Exhale slowly through your mouth for 11 seconds.

The reason this works is that breathing out longer than you breathe in sends a signal to your body that it's time to relax. It literally shifts your nervous system from "fight or flight" mode into a more relaxed state. Next time you're feeling the anxiety start to build, try 3 minutes of 7/11 breathing. I've used it in all kinds of stressful situations—work, social events, and, of course, when the IBS panic sets in.

If you would like to learn more, I highly recommend watching this talk by Dr. Alan Watkins:

Dr. Alan Watkins Talk Part 1 / Dr. Alan Watkins Talk Part 2

Tip #7: Use Rhythmic Breathing Techniques

Try it for yourself. Practise these breathing exercises for a few minutes each day, and especially when you feel anxiety creeping in. It won't magically solve all your problems, but it can help you approach stressful situations from a calmer, more positive state.

Negative Automatic Thoughts (NATs)

Breathing exercises can help calm your body, but what about your mind? This is where we need to talk about **Negative Automatic Thoughts (NATs)**. Before I received cognitive behavioural therapy (CBT), I didn't even realise how much my NATs controlled my life—how I thought, how I went about my day, and of course, how they affected my IBS. It was eye-opening to discover that many of my reactions were driven by unconscious, knee-jerk thoughts that happened so quickly I barely noticed them. These NATs were shaping my emotions and, in turn, my physical symptoms.

NATs are those automatic negative thoughts that creep in when you're stressed or anxious. They happen so fast that we often don't realise the impact they have until we're already feeling the emotional and physical consequences. For me, they would often sound like, *"What if I have a flare-up during this meeting?"* or *"I'll never get better."* At the time, I thought these were just worries I had to live with, but I soon learned that they were actually feeding into my anxiety and making my IBS worse.

For many people with IBS, the mind can be a powerful trigger. A single negative thought can send your body into stress mode, which directly affects your gut. This is where the gut-brain axis comes into play again. When your mind perceives stress, it signals your gut to prepare for a fight-or-flight response, which often leads to bloating, cramping, or urgency.

Learning to recognise and challenge my NATs through CBT was a turning point for me. It helped me see how my thoughts were fueling my stress and IBS, and gave me the tools to stop those thoughts from taking over. Managing your thoughts is just as important as managing your diet and lifestyle. By identifying and working with these NATs, you can start to break the cycle and regain control over your symptoms.

***

What is CBT and How Can It Help?

Cognitive Behavioural Therapy (CBT) is a well-known and widely-used approach for managing anxiety, stress, and negative thought patterns. It focuses on the link between your thoughts, feelings, and behaviours, and how they all influence each other. For someone like me, with IBS, learning CBT was a real eye-opener because it wasn't just about my symptoms—it was about how my thoughts were contributing to them.

CBT is all about identifying those unhelpful, automatic thoughts (the ones we often don't even realise we're having), questioning them, and then replacing them with more balanced and realistic ones. It's practical and action-oriented, which is exactly what I needed. Instead of feeling overwhelmed by negative thoughts, CBT helped me challenge them and take back control.

For example, if you're thinking *"I'll definitely have a flare-up at this event,"* CBT teaches you to ask yourself, *"Is there actual evidence for that? Or am I jumping to conclusions?"* By doing this, you can start to shift your thinking and reduce the stress that triggers IBS symptoms.

CBT is especially effective for those of us with IBS because it can break that vicious cycle where stress worsens your symptoms, and then those symptoms increase your stress. It's not about eliminating stress completely, but about managing your mind's response to it, which can make a world of difference when it comes to your gut.

Common Types of Negative Automatic Thoughts

Once I started learning about **Negative Automatic Thoughts (NATs)**, I realised just how often they were popping into my head, and how damaging they could be. These are the types of thoughts that happen so quickly, we don't even notice them, but they can have a huge impact on how we feel and, ultimately, on our IBS symptoms.

Here are some of the most common types of NATs I encountered, and maybe you'll recognise a few too:

- **Catastrophizing**: This is when you immediately jump to the worst-case scenario. It's that *"I'll never get better"* thought that pops up when symptoms flare. A classic example might be if you've got a big presentation coming up, and instead of thinking, *"I'll do my best,"* your mind goes to *"I'm going to mess this up completely, everyone will notice, and I'll look like a failure."* Your brain is convinced that one small mistake will lead to disaster, even though it's probably far from the truth. I was a massive catastrophizer. My mind absolutely loved doing it, and it took me a while to tame these thoughts—but it's worth putting in the effort.

- **Black-and-White Thinking**: This is when you see everything in extremes, with no middle ground. You make one mistake or have one bad day, and suddenly you're thinking, *"I messed up this diet plan, so I'll never manage my IBS."* Similarly, at work, if you make a small error during a presentation, you might think, *"I'm terrible at my job."* There's no room for a middle ground, and setbacks—whether with your health or career—feel permanent and overwhelming.

- **Mind Reading**: This one is sneaky. It's when you assume you know what others are thinking. For example, you might tell yourself, *"They must think I'm weak for having these IBS symptoms,"* when you can't really know that. Or in a meeting, if someone glances at their phone, you might think,

"They must be bored and think my presentation is awful," even though there's no real evidence for it. You're jumping to conclusions without any proof.

- **Fortune Telling**: This is when you predict the future without any solid evidence. For instance, you have a social event coming up and start thinking, *"I'll definitely have an IBS flare-up at that event,"* even though you can't possibly know for sure. Similarly, let's say you're going to an event—you might think, *"No one's going to talk to me, and I'll end up standing alone all night,"* even though there's no real basis for that assumption. Your mind is creating a negative outcome before anything even happens.

- **Overgeneralization**: This is when you draw a broad conclusion based on a single event. Let's say you have one particularly bad flare-up after trying a new food. You might think, *"I can't eat anything without getting sick,"* even though it was just one incident. Similarly, if you're late to work once, you might conclude, *"I'm always a failure,"* even though it was just an isolated situation. Overgeneralization makes it feel like a single setback defines your entire experience.

- **Personalisation**: This happens when you assume that other people's behaviour or reactions are a direct result of something you did, even when there's no evidence. For example, if a colleague seems quiet or distracted, you might think, *"They don't like me; it must be because of something I said,"* even though their mood could have nothing to do with you. Or, in an IBS context, you might think, *"They're annoyed with me because I keep having to go to the toilet all the time,"* even though there's no real evidence to support that assumption.

- **Emotional Reasoning**: This is when you assume that just because you feel something, it must be true. If you're feeling anxious or stressed, you might think, *"I'm failing,"* or *"I'm not capable,"* even though your emotions don't reflect the actual situation. A common IBS example might be, *"I feel sick, so I must be getting worse,"* when it's actually just temporary discomfort. Similarly, if you feel nervous about giving a presentation, you might think, *"I'm going to mess it up,"* even though you've prepared well and can handle it.

To be honest, I was guilty of nearly all of these NATs. They are really detrimental to your health- mental and physical. I know these kinds of thoughts feel real, but they're often just patterns that keep us stuck in a cycle of stress and anxiety. The good news is, once you recognise them, you can start to challenge them and stop them from taking over.

Creating Alternative Automatic Thoughts

Once you've identified your **Negative Automatic Thoughts (NATs)**, the next step is to challenge and replace them with more balanced, realistic alternatives. This is one of the most powerful tools I learned through CBT because it gave me a way to take back control of my mind, rather than letting it run wild with negative thoughts that only fueled my stress and worsened my IBS symptoms.

For example, if your NAT is something like, *"I'll never get better,"* you can challenge it by asking yourself questions like: *"Is that really true? What evidence do I have to support that? Is there another way to look at this?"*. Often, you'll find that your NAT isn't as grounded in reality as you initially thought, and there's usually a more balanced, alternative thought you can adopt.

The goal isn't to dismiss your feelings, but to see things more clearly and reduce the emotional intensity that comes with NATs. This process works not only for IBS-related thoughts but also for everyday stressors and challenges.

Here's how you can create **Alternative Automatic Thoughts**:

1. **Recognise the NAT**: Catch the negative thought as it pops up. It could be triggered by a stressful situation, a symptom, or an interaction with someone. This is the first step in breaking the cycle.

2. **Challenge the Thought**: Ask yourself if this thought is really true. Is there evidence that supports it? Is there evidence that contradicts it? Could there be another explanation? Often, the NAT doesn't stand up to scrutiny once you start to examine it more closely.

3. **Create an Alternative Thought**: Once you've challenged the NAT, create a more balanced and realistic alternative thought. This thought should reflect a calmer, more rational response to the situation and help you feel more in control.

Let's break this down into a few examples using a table to show how NATs can be replaced with **Alternative Thoughts**:

Negative Automatic Thought (NAT)	Alternative Thought
"I'll never get better."	"I've had good days before, so I know I'm capable of improvement."
"I'm going to have a flare-up at the event."	"I've managed events before, and I have tools to help me if I feel uncomfortable."
"They must think I'm weak for having IBS symptoms."	"I can't know what they're thinking, and it's likely they're focused on their own concerns."
"I messed up that presentation, so I'm bad at my job."	"I made one mistake, but I did well in other parts of the presentation. I can improve next time."
"No one will talk to me at this social event."	"I've been to events before where I've connected with others. I can take it one conversation at a time."
"I'm always going to feel this bloated."	"This bloating has passed before, and I can take steps to ease it again."
"If I try this new food, my IBS will flare up."	"I can try a small portion first, and I've handled new foods before with success."
"My colleagues think I'm not capable because I struggle with stress."	"I can't know what they're thinking, and my performance in other tasks has been strong."

Negative Automatic Thought (NAT)	Alternative Thought
"I'll never be able to stick to this diet plan."	"I've had slip-ups before but was able to get back on track. I can adjust and try again."
"I didn't finish my task on time, so I'm terrible at managing my work."	"I missed a deadline this time, but I've met deadlines before and can improve my time management."
"If I make a mistake in this meeting, everyone will think I'm incompetent."	"One mistake won't define me—people understand that everyone slips up occasionally."
"I'll never be able to control my anxiety."	"I've managed my anxiety before, and I have tools that can help me cope."
"This argument is going to ruin my relationship."	"We've had disagreements before, and we've always managed to work through them."

These alternative thoughts provide a more balanced perspective and help reduce the emotional impact of the original NATs. By practising this process regularly—just like strengthening a muscle—you'll find it easier to shift your thinking in the moment. The more you challenge your NATs, the more automatic this process will become, helping you feel more in control of your thoughts and emotions.

Challenging and Replacing a NAT

Let's walk through a deeper example to see this process in action:

1. **Situation**: You have a work presentation coming up, and your IBS has been flaring up recently.
2. **NAT**: *"I'm going to have a flare-up during my presentation, and everyone will think I'm unprofessional."*
3. **Challenging the NAT**: Ask yourself, *"Is there evidence that this will definitely happen? Have I handled presentations before? What steps can I take to prepare and manage my symptoms?"*
4. **Alternative Thought**: *"I've handled presentations in the past, and I have strategies in place to manage my symptoms. Even if I feel uncomfortable, I can take a break if I need to."*

This process helps reduce the anxiety tied to the situation by challenging the negative thought and replacing it with something more grounded and realistic. Whether it's an IBS-related thought or a more general stressor, this technique can help you reframe your thinking and manage your stress.

Why This Practice Matters

By practising this regularly, you'll start to notice how much more in control you feel over your thoughts, emotions, and, as a result, your physical well-being. **Negative Automatic Thoughts** can fuel stress, anxiety, and even IBS symptoms, but by challenging them and replacing them with balanced alternatives, you're taking the first steps toward creating a healthier, more positive mindset.

Tip #8: Challenge Negative Thoughts

Identify and reframe negative automatic thoughts. Replace them with balanced, realistic thoughts to break the cycle of stress and physical symptoms.

***

Visualisation: Shifting Focus

Another really effective tool for breaking the anxiety-symptom cycle is visualisation. It might seem odd at first—how can simply imagining something in your mind make your gut feel better? But it's surprisingly powerful. Visualisation works because it helps redirect your focus away from your anxiety and symptoms, and towards something calming and peaceful.

Here's how to get started:

1. **Step 1: Choose a Calming Image**
   Find a mental image that brings you peace. It could be a beach, a forest, a cosy room—whatever makes you feel at ease.

2. **Step 2: Engage Your Senses**

   Picture this place in vivid detail. Imagine the sounds, smells, and sensations. How does the sand feel under your feet? What does the air smell like? Engaging your senses helps immerse your mind in the image, shifting your attention away from your anxious thoughts.

3. **Step 3: Breathe Into the Image**

   While you're visualising this peaceful place, breathe slowly and deeply. For example, inhale for 4 seconds, hold for 4, and exhale for 4 (this even ratio is called box breathing). Focus on the image and your breath simultaneously, letting your body settle into calmness. Below are some links to help with this:

- Visualisation Meditation
- 10-Minute Guided Visualisation for Anxiety

Grounding: Bringing Yourself Back to the Present

Grounding techniques help you stay present in the moment and pull you out of spiralling anxious thoughts. One method I've found particularly useful is the **5-4-3-2-1 technique**. It engages your senses and brings your attention back to the physical world around you, helping break the cycle of anxiety. This is especially effective if you're suddenly anxious or nervous about something. I usually do this before a breathing exercise.

Here's how it works:

1. **Name 5 things you can see**
   Look around you and identify five things you can see. It could be anything—your laptop, a tree outside, the pattern on a carpet.

2. **Name 4 things you can feel**
   Bring your awareness to touch. Notice the texture of your clothes, the temperature of the air, or the sensation of your feet on the ground.

3. **Name 3 things you can hear**
   Focus on the sounds around you. It could be distant traffic, birds chirping, or the hum of an appliance.

4. **Name 2 things you can smell**
   Take in the smells around you. This one can be trickier, but even the smell of your soap or the fresh air counts.

5. **Name 1 thing you can taste**
   If possible, focus on a taste in your mouth. If you can't taste anything, simply think of a flavour you enjoy, like your favourite food.

The **5-4-3-2-1 technique** is quick and simple, yet very effective at shifting your focus back to the present moment and calming your mind. You can use it whenever anxiety starts creeping in, and it works particularly well when you feel your IBS symptoms starting to flare.

***

Acupuncture: A Possible Path to Relief?

When you're dealing with IBS, you'll try almost anything to get some relief. That's exactly how I ended up trying acupuncture. In Korea, where I was living at the time, acupuncture is a big part of traditional medicine known as *Hanyak*. It's everywhere, and people swear by it for all kinds of ailments—so I thought, why not give it a go? What's the worst that could happen, right?

Walking into the clinic, I was already a bit on edge. I was the only foreigner in the room, and the idea of having needles stuck in my stomach and back didn't exactly calm my nerves. But I figured, if this has been working for centuries, there must be something to it.

The Research on Acupuncture for IBS

Turns out, there's actually some scientific backing to acupuncture for IBS. Studies suggest it can help regulate gut motility (the speed at which food moves through your system), reduce visceral hypersensitivity (basically, that super-sensitive pain you feel in your gut), and even affect the gut-brain axis, which is crucial for managing stress-induced IBS symptoms.

For example, research[1] published in *The American Journal of Gastroenterology* found that acupuncture led to real improvements in bloating and bowel regularity.

Another review[2] that combined results from several studies found it can help with abdominal pain and improve the quality of life for people with IBS. However, even the researchers admit that more studies are needed to get the full picture.

---

1. Lembo, A. J., Conboy, L., Kelley, J. M., et al. (2012). Acupuncture for irritable bowel syndrome: A randomized controlled trial. *The American Journal of Gastroenterology, 107*(6), 903–911. https://doi.org/10.1038/ajg.2012.113

2. MacPherson, H, Tilbrook, H, Bland, M, Tilbrook, H, Spackman, E, & Torgerson, D (2014). Acupuncture for irritable bowel syndrome: A systematic review and meta-analysis. *World Journal of Gastroenterology, 20*(6), 1871–1877. https://doi.org/10.3748/wjg.v20.i6.1871

My Personal Experience with Acupuncture

For me, though, acupuncture didn't quite hit the mark. I went through a few sessions, but my IBS symptoms didn't really budge. Looking back, I can't help but wonder if it had more to do with my mindset. I wasn't exactly in the most relaxed state—nervous about being the only foreigner in the room, surrounded by needles in my gut. I was already anxious, which is never a great start for something that's supposed to help you relax.

But I also think my scepticism played a role. I didn't go in expecting it to work, and maybe that's why it didn't. The mind-body connection is powerful, and sometimes what you believe can influence the outcome more than you think.

The Role of Expectations

This ties directly into what we talked about earlier—the "Expectation Effect." Research has shown that what you believe going into a treatment can play a huge role in how well it works. The same applies to acupuncture. If you go into it thinking, "This might help," your body is more likely to respond positively. Some studies show that acupuncture has real, measurable benefits, but how you approach it mentally can make all the difference. If you're open to it and expect a good result, you may very well see one. On the flip side, scepticism and anxiety, like what I experienced during my sessions, might hold you back from seeing the full potential of the treatment.

Should You Try Acupuncture?

So, is it worth trying acupuncture for your IBS? It's generally safe and might work for some people, even though it didn't for me. If you're curious about it and have access to a good practitioner, it could be worth a shot. Just go in with an open mind and remember that with IBS, it's all about finding what works for you.

While acupuncture didn't solve my IBS, that doesn't mean it won't work for you. Everyone's experience is different, and this might just be the needle in the haystack you were looking for.

***

Being in Nature – Forest Bathing

Ever notice how a walk in the park or time spent outdoors can instantly lift your mood? There's a reason for that. "Forest bathing," a Japanese practice known as *shinrin-yoku*, (because everything sounds better in Japanese) involves immersing yourself in nature, soaking in the sights, sounds, and smells of the forest. It's more than just a walk; it's about truly being present, grounding yourself, and reconnecting with the natural world. Studies have shown that spending time in nature can significantly reduce anxiety, improve mood, and even lower cortisol levels (the stress hormone).

And you don't need a forest to get these benefits—any green space will do. A simple walk in a nearby park, sitting under a tree, or even tending to your garden can work wonders. Stepping away from screens, letting go of daily stresses, and allowing nature to do its calming magic can be a perfect addition to your toolkit for managing stress and IBS.

I've been lucky enough to live on the edge of a forest, and as often as I can, in the morning, I take a 15-minute walk through the trees. It's a small ritual that has transformed my day—calming my mind and setting a positive tone. It's funny because when I was a kid, my parents would make the whole family hike somewhere around the Peak District, and I distinctly remember resenting that and finding it pointless - going up the hill only to come back down again. It's only now, as an adult, that I really realise and appreciate the power of being in nature. And on the days when I can't make it out for my walk, my body immediately senses the difference—more tension, less focus. So now, whenever I can, I escape to the countryside; it feels like it's cleansing my soul and helps to find inner peace. Nature definitely has a way of resetting my mind and grounding me in a way that nothing else can. Try it!

In case you can't go to a forest or a park near you, I even find the forest bathing videos really relaxing too. Give this video a try:

Shinrin-Yoku, (Forest Bathing)

Meditation: Calm Your Mind, Calm Your Gut

Let's face it—meditation has gone from being something "weird" to a mainstream tool for improving mental health. You've probably heard about its benefits for stress, anxiety, and focus. But what you may not realise is that meditation can also help with IBS by giving you more control over your thoughts and reactions.

For years, I simply just didn't believe in it. I thought, *"How is sitting quietly going to help my stomach problems?"* But when I finally tried it, the difference was clear. Meditation taught me to stop treating every little twinge in my gut like a disaster. It allowed me to let go of anxious, negative thoughts that were fueling my symptoms.

One of the most helpful techniques I discovered was imagining my thoughts as taxis passing by on the street. I stand on the sidewalk, watching them drive past. But sometimes, without realising it, I find myself inside one of those taxis—caught up in a thought. When that happens, instead of panicking, I gently step back out, return to the sidewalk, and let the taxis continue passing by. The goal is to remain the observer, without judgement, and calmly bring yourself back to the present.

If that doesn't quite work for you, let's go a bit deeper with another analogy. Imagine yourself sitting on the ground, watching the sky above. Your thoughts are like clouds—some are light and fluffy, others dark and stormy. But the key is to realise that, just like clouds, thoughts come and go. They don't define the sky, and they don't define you.

By practising this perspective, you gain more control over how you respond to those thoughts, rather than letting them control you.

This separation is essential for managing stress and anxiety, which are known triggers for IBS symptoms. When you can observe your thoughts without judgement or attachment, you create a mental "buffer." This buffer allows you to respond more calmly to situations that might normally cause stress, fostering emotional regulation that extends to your body. The calming effects can directly promote better gut health, helping you navigate life's challenges with more ease and resilience.

So, each time you meditate or practise mindful breathing, remember that your goal isn't to stop thoughts from coming, but simply to observe them as they pass—much like watching clouds in the sky. This is where the magic happens, as you start to separate yourself from the noise and discover a calmer, more balanced state of mind and body.

Here's a simple guide to getting started with meditation:

1. **Find a comfortable seat**. Sit on the floor or in a chair with your back straight and hips slightly tilted forward. This posture will help keep you alert but relaxed. Trust me—if you're slouched, it's all too easy to drift off!

2. **Set an intention**. Why are you meditating today? Taking a moment to clarify this purpose helps ground your practice, guiding your focus and adding meaning to each session.

3. **Focus on your breath**. Notice the air moving in and out of

your nostrils. Don't try to control it—just become aware of it.

4. **Catch wandering thoughts**. Your mind will inevitably drift—especially when you're new to meditation. Don't get frustrated; this is all part of the process. Each time you catch yourself thinking, view it as a small win. Every moment of awareness strengthens your practice, like building mental muscles one thought at a time. Gently bring your focus back to your breath (or whatever anchor you've chosen, like taxis or clouds drifting by).

5. **Count your breaths**. Each inhale or exhale counts individually; go up to 10, then start over. But remember, the goal isn't to reach 10—it's the act of counting that helps you stay focused. Sometimes, you may count beyond 10 or need to start back at 1 when your mind wanders, and that's perfectly okay. If a thought comes up, gently bring your attention back and start from 1 again. At first, you might rarely reach 10 without drifting off, but with patience, it becomes easier—and it's worth it. If you feel ready, you can transition to focusing solely on your breath without counting, but I recommend trying this later on or in the final part of your meditation.

6. **Aim for 15-20 minutes**. You don't need to meditate for hours; even 10-20 minutes a day can make a noticeable difference in how you feel. If you're just starting, begin with 5 minutes a day to ease into the practice. Building this new

habit is what matters most, so starting small and gradually increasing your time is the best approach.

Resources to Help You Get Started:

There are countless videos now for Meditation. So, find one that works for you. In the past, I found a YouTube channel called **Mindah-Lee Kumar (The Enthusiastic Buddhist)** incredibly helpful, especially when starting out. Check out this video: Mindfulness Meditation Breathing Exercises

Other useful apps I've used include:

- **Headspace** – A great app with hundreds of meditation videos and programs to guide you. For me, Headspace was perfect for those "emergency moments" when I needed a quick tool to calm down. Its guided practices are easy to follow, especially if you're feeling overwhelmed and need help quickly.

- **Calm** – Offers meditation programs as well as relaxing stories and sounds. I used Calm a lot for sleep—it has some fantastic bedtime stories and relaxing music to drift off to, though I've stopped using it lately. It's particularly great if you're looking for something to unwind at night.

- **Happier** (formerly **10% Happier**) – This one is my all-time favourite. Based on Dan Harris' approach, it's practical and no-nonsense, which I found refreshing. However, full disclaimer: I read his book "10% Happier", so I might be a little biased! It's a bit pricier, but I always thought it was worth it for the relatable and straightforward take on meditation.

Tip #9: Try Meditation and Relaxation Techniques

Give meditation a chance for two weeks, even if you think you're not the "meditation type." Trust me, it's worth the effort. Once you get the hang of it, you'll find it not only helps manage your IBS symptoms but also makes you feel a lot calmer in everyday life.

***

Autogenic Relaxation Techniques

I learned this technique from a healthcare practitioner. At first, I was a bit uncertain (like a lot of these new techniques), but I kept an open mind. This is important when trying new things—just give them a go, and if they don't work, move on. Autogenic relaxation is a mind-body practice designed to bring about a sense of calm and ease. Unlike other techniques we've covered, this approach uses gentle self-suggestion to invoke feelings of warmth, heaviness, and calm throughout your body. It's like nudging your mind to let go of stress and tension—perfect for soothing both your nerves and gut.

Autogenic relaxation helps calm the autonomic nervous system, balancing out the stress response (the "fight-or-flight" mode) that often wreaks havoc on digestion. Unlike breathing techniques, which focus on regulating breath to quickly activate the parasympathetic nervous system, autogenic relaxation uses visualisation and self-suggestion to reach a deeper state of calmness. While breathing techniques provide quick relief by focusing on rhythm, autogenic relaxation guides you through mental imagery and affirmations to create sensations of heaviness and warmth. Both are effective in different ways and together, they can be powerful tools for managing IBS.

What is Autogenic Relaxation?

Autogenic relaxation is a self-guided method that uses visualisation and repetition to achieve a state of calm. Developed by German psychiatrist Johannes Schultz, it involves focusing on sensations like heaviness, warmth, and ease through simple, repeated phrases. The goal is to tap into your body's natural ability to self-regulate, almost like a gentle form of self-hypnosis. For IBS sufferers, this technique can ease tension in the gut and support better digestive health.

How to Practise Autogenic Relaxation

You can do autogenic relaxation anywhere—at home, at work, or even while travelling.

Here's how:

1. **Preparation**: Find a quiet, comfortable space where you won't be disturbed. Sit or lie down, loosen any tight clothing, and close your eyes.

2. **Focusing on Heaviness**: Start by creating a sense of heaviness in your limbs. Use phrases like: *"My right arm is heav y... My left arm is heavy... Both arms are heavy..."* Gradually move through your body, letting a wave of heaviness help your muscles relax.

3. **Focusing on Warmth**: Shift to a sensation of warmth: *"My right arm is warm... My left arm is warm... Both arms are warm..."* Extend this warmth through your entire body as if you're basking in gentle sunlight.

4. **Breathing and Heartbeat Awareness**: Bring attention to your breath and heartbeat, keeping them gentle and calm: *"My breathing is calm and steady... My heartbeat is regular and even..."* Let this rhythm soothe you, like a lullaby.

5. **Overall Body Relaxation**: End by guiding warmth and calmness to your whole body: *"My abdomen feels warm and at ease... My whole body is deeply relaxed..."*

If you're new to autogenic relaxation, starting with an audio/video guide can help. Here are some options to try:

- Autogenic Relaxation Guide
- Short Guided Relaxation
- Body Relaxation Script

A Guided Script to Get Started

Here's a quick guide for a short session:

- "My arms are heavy and warm..."
- "My legs are relaxed, heavy, and warm..."
- "My breathing is calm and natural..."

- "My heartbeat is steady and relaxed..."
- "My abdomen is warm, and my whole body feels deeply relaxed..."

When and How to Use Autogenic Relaxation

- **Daily Practice**: Begin with 5-10 minutes a day, increasing to about 20 minutes if it feels beneficial. Try to practise at consistent times, such as before bed or after work.
- **Situational Use**: Use autogenic relaxation whenever anxiety or stress hits. Whether facing a stressful presentation, feeling overwhelmed, or dealing with IBS discomfort, this technique can ground and relax you.

Tips for Success

- **Start Slowly**: It's normal for autogenic relaxation to feel unfamiliar at first. Start with short sessions and build up as you grow more comfortable.
- **Don't Force It**: If feeling "heavy" or "warm" doesn't come easily, don't worry. The aim is gentle practice, not perfection.
- **Practise Regularly**: Consistency is key. Studies show that

it is most effective when it's done regularly. So try and make autogenic relaxation a part of your daily routine.

- **Be Patient with Yourself**: Some days will be easier than others. Each session is a step toward cultivating calmness.

Final Thoughts

Autogenic relaxation is like hitting a "reset" button for your body and mind—a low-effort way to tap into your relaxation response and regain control over stress-induced IBS symptoms. With regular practice, you'll find it easier to reach a state of calm for both your mind and gut. So carve out a few minutes each day, find a quiet corner, and give yourself permission to relax. You might be surprised at how effective this gentle practice can be for your overall well-being.

As we've explored various techniques like breathing exercises and meditation, managing anxiety becomes key to breaking the IBS-stress cycle. If you're looking for a bit more structure to specifically manage anxiety, I highly recommend a free **30-day anxiety course** on YouTube that helped me immensely.

The course offers short, daily videos with practical techniques like breathing, visualisation, and reframing negative thoughts—all of which align perfectly with what you're learning here. It's an easy way to deepen your practice and stay consistent. You can check it out here: 30-Day Anxiety Course on YouTube (QR code)

Breaking Free from the Loop

IBS doesn't have to control your life. The cycle of anxiety and symptoms may seem relentless, but tools like 7/11 breathing, visualisation, self-affirmations, and meditation can help you start to break that loop. Remember, progress takes practice and patience—it won't happen overnight. The real power lies in consistent small steps. Each time you use these techniques, you're retraining your body and mind to respond more calmly and positively. Over time, you'll notice a shift: more moments of peace, fewer flares of panic, and a greater sense of control over your symptoms.

It's so bloody easy to not do any of these techniques and just go about your day. I know because I was there. I really need you to get yourself trying these techniques, start with one for a week and see how it goes. The most important thing to remember is that every effort counts. The anxiety-symptom loop may seem daunting, but it's not unbreakable. Every deep breath, every moment spent visualising calm, and every positive affirmation (see below) is a step toward reclaiming your well-being. You'll find that as you practise these techniques, the fear of symptoms holds less power over you. Each day, you are learning to step back from that cliff, breathe, and find your balance. And with that balance, life with IBS becomes not just manageable but a journey you can navigate with confidence and self-compassion. Keep going!

Now that you've explored the ways anxiety and negative thoughts fuel your IBS symptoms, it's time to take a closer look at your own thinking patterns. Noticing your Negative Automatic Thoughts (NATs) is the first step in breaking their control over your mind and body. These thoughts often pop up unnoticed, but once you become aware of them, they lose some of their power. By practising reframing those thoughts, you can start to shift your mindset and see improvements in both your anxiety and IBS symptoms.

***

The Power of Positive Affirmations

I'll be honest: when I first came across the idea of positive affirmations, I felt pretty strange saying them. They seemed cheesy, and a big part of me doubted they'd actually work. I remember being introduced to the concept in my early 20s through the book *Feel the Fear and Do It Anyway*. The idea of standing there, repeating phrases like "I'm in control of my body" or "My gut is calm," felt downright embarrassing. In fact, I didn't tell anyone I was doing it—I kept it my little secret, especially because I was using these affirmations during some of the most turbulent and difficult times in my life.

But something shifted for me. Like with a lot of these things, I realised that if I went into the process already thinking it wouldn't work, I was setting myself up for failure. I had to give it a real shot. So, I decided to keep an open mind and just try it out—if it didn't work, I could always move on. But allowing myself to believe it might actually help was key. The consistency and belief I applied to these affirmations made all the difference for me. I was genuinely surprised at how useful they became, and that's why I'm dedicating an entire section to them in this book. Don't knock them until you've tried it!

Positive affirmations can be a powerful tool in reinforcing the mind-body connection, especially for managing IBS symptoms. They remind your mind to send the right signals to your gut, promoting relaxation and control over discomfort. However, their effectiveness largely depends on two things: belief and consistency. If you don't believe in the affirmations or feel disconnected from the words you're saying, the results will likely be limited. But when you approach affirmations with an open mind, they can become a helpful tool in cultivating a healthier mindset and well-being.

What Are Positive Affirmations?

At their core, positive affirmations are short, positive statements designed to challenge negative thoughts and encourage more optimistic thinking. The goal is to influence the subconscious mind, shaping your mindset in a way that reinforces self-empowerment. When practised regularly, affirmations can create new mental pathways, helping to cultivate a healthier relationship with your thoughts and emotions.

When it comes to managing IBS, the connection between the mind and body is critical. Your gut and brain are constantly communicating, so the way you think and feel can have a direct impact on your physical symptoms. This is where positive affirmations come into play—they help shift the mind into a more relaxed, confident state, which in turn, calms the body's physical responses, including those in the gut.

How Affirmations Can Help IBS

So, how do affirmations help with something as complex as IBS? It all comes down to the gut-brain axis again! When you're stressed, your brain sends signals to your gut that can trigger symptoms like cramping, bloating, or urgency. Positive affirmations help to counteract those negative signals by promoting a more relaxed and controlled mindset. When you reinforce calm, your body begins to mirror that state, which can ease gut-related discomfort.

Affirmations aren't a magic cure, but they are a tool that can help retrain the way your mind interacts with your body. By consistently repeating affirmations focused on gut health and relaxation, you can support the healing process by calming your nervous system and reducing stress.

Examples of Affirmations for Gut Health

Here are some affirmations that can help foster a sense of calm and control over IBS symptoms:

- “My body knows how to heal, and I trust the process.”
- “My gut is at ease, working in harmony with my mind.”
- “I release tension from my gut, and my digestion flows smoothly.”
- “With each breath, my gut becomes calmer and more relaxed.”
- “I nourish my body with peace, and it responds with comfort.”
- “I am in control of my body, and my gut responds with balance and health.”
- “Each day, my gut feels stronger and more settled.”
- “I am safe, relaxed, and my gut is free from discomfort.”
- “My gut is a healthy, well-functioning part of me.”
- “I am calm, and my body follows this calmness with ease.”

These affirmations reinforce the mind-body connection, promoting relaxation and control over gut-related discomfort. You can choose a few that resonate most with you or create your own personalised affirmations that align with your specific needs.

Personalising Your Affirmations

One of the most important aspects of using affirmations is making sure they feel personal and relevant to your situation. You can absolutely take the affirmations I've shared and use them as-is, but you'll find them more powerful if you adapt them to your own voice and needs.

When creating your own affirmations, keep them positive, in the present tense, and focused on outcomes that you genuinely want to achieve. For example, instead of saying, "I don't want to feel pain," reframe it as, "My gut feels calm and at ease." The key is to focus on what you *do* want, rather than what you want to avoid.

How to Use Affirmations Effectively

Affirmations work best when they're practised consistently. Here's a simple routine you can follow to make them a regular part of your day:

- **Morning Affirmations:** Start your day by repeating your chosen affirmations while brushing your teeth or getting ready for work. This sets a positive tone for the day ahead.
- **During Meditation:** After you have started meditating for a while, incorporate your affirmations into your practice. As you focus on your breath, repeat the affirmations in your mind.

- **Before Bed:** End your day with a calming affirmation, reminding yourself that your body is healing and working in harmony while you rest.

A helpful tip: It's easy to forget to practise affirmations, especially when life gets busy. Setting an alarm on your phone can be a great way to remind yourself throughout the day. Just a quick reminder 3 times a day will help you stay consistent and build the habit over time. Without a nudge, it's easy to let the day slip by and forget to do them altogether.

You can also combine affirmations with visualisation for an added boost. For example, while saying "My gut is calm and relaxed," you can imagine a peaceful river gently flowing through your digestive system, bringing balance and ease.

Overcoming Doubt or Resistance

I completely get it—affirmations can feel strange at first. There's a part of you that might roll your eyes or doubt whether saying a few positive phrases can really make a difference. I felt the **exact** same way. But here's the thing: if you go into it thinking it won't work, it probably won't. Belief is a big part of the process.

So, I encourage you to push past the initial scepticism and give it a try. Start with just one or two affirmations that resonate with you, and say them regularly for a few weeks. Keep an open mind and watch for subtle shifts in how you feel. Remember, affirmations are just one tool in your IBS management toolkit, but they can be a powerful one when used consistently.

Why Affirmations Matter

At the end of the day, affirmations are about more than just positive thinking—they're about reshaping the way you communicate with your body. By repeating affirmations that focus on health, calm, and healing, you're sending signals to your body that support the gut-brain connection. It's not a quick fix, but over time, affirmations can help foster a healthier, more balanced mindset that makes managing IBS a little easier.

So, don't knock it until you try it! You might just find that these simple phrases have more power than you thought.

Reflection and Practical Step

Your Negative Automatic Thoughts (NATs)

Negative Automatic Thoughts (NATs) can intensify stress and IBS symptoms, creating a cycle that feels difficult to break. Recognising and reframing these thoughts can help shift your mindset, making it easier to manage symptoms. This section will guide you in identifying and challenging your NATs to create a calmer and more balanced mental environment.

Exercise: Reflection on Your NATs

Prompt: Take some time to reflect on the types of Negative Automatic Thoughts (NATs) you tend to have when your IBS symptoms flare up. Do you catastrophize, overgeneralise, or engage in black-and-white thinking? Write down a few examples of your common NATs and how they impact your stress levels and gut health. Next, create alternative thoughts to challenge those NATs, using the examples from this chapter to help. For instance, if your NAT is, "I'll never feel better," try reframing it to, "I've had good days before, and I can have them again."

Practical Step: Gradual Introduction of Mindfulness, Breathing, and Relaxation Techniques

Incorporating mindfulness practices into your routine can help you manage your symptoms by calming both your mind and body. However, with so many practical techniques here, this section offers a straightforward, three-week plan to integrate them at a relaxed pace. Tackling everything at once can feel overwhelming—let's be honest, it's easy to end up doing none of it! By trying just a few techniques each week, you'll discover what really works for you, build lasting habits, and start to feel the real benefits of each practice.

Week 1: Meditation, Breathing Practice, & Affirmations

Start by incorporating meditation, rhythmic breathing, and positive affirmations together.

- **Meditation**: Try a short meditation practice for 5-10 minutes each day. Find a comfortable spot, focus on your breath, and allow yourself to relax. Use a guided meditation or simply focus on each inhale and exhale. Create a habit by pairing it with an existing routine. For example, meditate after having a cup of tea when you come home from work.

- **Rhythmic Breathing**: Practise 7/11 breathing—inhale for 7 seconds, and exhale for 11 seconds. Adjust the ratio (e.g., 4/6, 5/8) depending on what feels natural. Pair this with your meditation or do it when you feel stress rising, like before breakfast or during a work break. Set a reminder for before lunch to practise this as well.

- **Affirmations**: While you're practising meditation or rhythmic breathing, add in some positive affirmations to reinforce calm and control. For example, say or think, "My gut is calm and relaxed," or "I am in control of my body's response." You can also repeat affirmations in moments of stress, pairing them with your breathing exercises for a soothing effect. Or, try setting an alarm and doing them 3 times a day.

Week 2: Visualisation or Forest BathingPick one of the following to focus on during Week 2:

- **Visualisation**: Practise imagining a peaceful, calming scene when you feel anxious. Use one of the guides to help. Engage all your senses—imagine the sounds, sights, and smells of your safe space. Pair this with your breathing exercises for an added calming effect.

- **Forest Bathing**: Spend time in nature at least once a week. This could be a walk in the park or simply sitting outside. Focus on being present, letting the sights and sounds of nature help you relax. You'll notice a calming effect on both your mind and body. I like to walk along rivers and focus on the sound of the water.

Week 3: Autogenic Relaxation

- **Autogenic Relaxation**: Start by listening to a guided autogenic relaxation video. This method focuses on calming thoughts and sensations, like feeling warmth in your limbs or slowing your heartbeat. Once you're comfortable with the technique, you can try doing it by yourself. Lie down in a quiet space, focus on one part of your body at a time, and imagine warmth or relaxation spreading there. Practise this once or twice a day for the best results.

Final Tip: Building These Practices Into Your Routine

The key to success with these techniques is consistency. Start small, but make them a part of your daily routine. For example, you can practise rhythmic breathing before meals, meditation after work, and try autogenic relaxation before bed. By gradually introducing these practices, you'll find that they begin to feel more natural, and you'll notice a positive shift in your body's response to stress and IBS triggers.

Chapter 4

From Chaos to Calm: Tackling Internal Stress

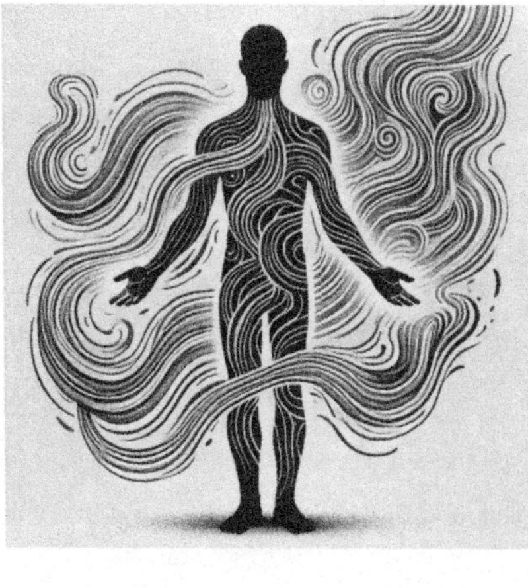

In the previous chapter, we explored how anxiety can trigger and worsen IBS symptoms, creating a vicious cycle. Stress comes at us from both within and outside—as an internal experience and an external influence—and each plays a role in how we cope with IBS. This chapter is all about breaking that cycle from the inside out, with tools to manage the inner stress and worry that take a toll on your body. Then, in Part 2, we'll shift our focus to tackle those outer stressors—like challenging situations, people, and environments that pile on the pressure. For now, let's jump into strategies that will help you calm your mind and body, equipping you to start from within.

***

Armour Your Mind

I remember listening to an Australian Buddhist monk many years ago—though his name slips my memory, the story he told, however, has stayed with me vividly. It was about a young king who once walked barefoot on his vast kingdom's scorching hot sand, blistering his feet with every painful step. Distressed by this suffering, the king decided that he would cover the entire kingdom with leather to protect his feet. But then, an advisor proposed a much simpler solution: instead of covering all the land with leather, why not just cover his own feet?

And so, the king wrapped his feet in leather, creating the world's first shoes.

This story hit me like a bolt of lightning, and I instantly knew what I had to do. Rather than trying to change everything around me—whether stressful situations, negative people, or external circumstances that were causing me distress—I needed to focus on wrapping my own mind in "leather." In other words, I had to learn how to protect my emotional well-being and inner peace from the inevitable challenges and stressors of life. And for anyone dealing with IBS, this idea of "armouring your mind" can be a transformative change.

The world is like that vast stretch of burning sand—it's chaotic, unpredictable, and sometimes harsh. But trying to change every stressful aspect of life is like trying to cover the entire kingdom in leather—it's simply not possible. What is possible, though, is changing how you experience and respond to the world. By wrapping your own mind in "leather," you develop a mental and emotional buffer, protecting your sense of calm and reducing the impact of stress and anxiety.

To "armour your mind" is to consciously cultivate resilience and inner strength. Just like the king who wrapped his feet, you can learn to navigate life without letting the "hot sand" burn you every step of the way. This doesn't mean ignoring or avoiding problems, but it does mean learning to respond to them with a greater sense of ease, calm, and emotional protection.

Practical Steps to "Armour Your Mind"

1. **Reframe Stressful Situations**

   Rather than focusing on how situations are "ruining" your day or contributing to your anxiety, ask yourself: "How can I respond to this differently?" or "What is within my control right now?" This shift in perspective helps you move from feeling overwhelmed to feeling empowered, allowing you to handle stress with more clarity and confidence.

2. **Set Emotional Boundaries**

   Just as you wouldn't let anyone step on your freshly polished leather shoes, don't allow others' negativity or opinions to invade your peace. Learn to recognise what's yours to carry emotionally and what belongs to others.

3. **Visualisation of Boundaries**

   Mentally visualise an emotional barrier between yourself and others. This could be a glass wall or a protective bubble that lets you engage with others but keeps their negative energy or emotions from overwhelming you. This technique weirdly works really well with me!

4. **Develop Self-Compassion**

   Wrap your mind in self-compassion. When you experience stress, rather than criticising yourself for not handling it perfectly, acknowledge that you are doing your best and extend kindness toward yourself. This kindness toward yourself serves as a mental shield, helping you recover from stress without adding self-judgement.

5. **Practise Mindfulness and Grounding Techniques**

   By focusing on the present moment and engaging in grounding exercises (like rhythmic breathing or observing your surroundings), you give your mind the "leather shoes" it needs to walk through the hot sand of life with less pain. Whether it's focusing on your senses through grounding or using rhythmic breathing to calm your mind, mindfulness helps centre you in moments of stress.

6. **The "STOP" Method**

   In moments of stress or emotional overwhelm, use the STOP method to regain control. If you practise this a few times, it works wonders and prevents a lot of heated arguments to be honest! Here it is:
   S: Stop what you're doing.
   T: Take a breath to centre yourself.
   O: Observe your emotions and physical sensations without judgement.
   P: Proceed mindfully, choosing how you want to respond, not react.

7. **Practise Emotional Regulation**

   Emotional regulation means learning how to recognise and control your emotions. When stress begins to rise, notice it without reacting impulsively. Acknowledge how you feel, and choose a calming strategy like rhythmic breathing or grounding. This prevents stress from snowballing and helps you respond in a more balanced way.

Tip #10: Build a Mental Armour

By implementing these practices, you can "armour your mind" against the daily stressors and challenges, creating a protective layer around your well-being, just like the king who learned to walk across the burning sands with ease.

***

Handling Stress

Handling stress is like training a puppy—hard at first, but eventually, you gain control, and it doesn't ruin the carpet (or your gut). If you've ever stayed up all night, mulling over a problem that still isn't solved by morning, then welcome to the club. We've all been there. But here's the trick: breaking that thought spiral. Reframing stressful situations as opportunities, using visualisation, grounding techniques, and journaling can act like leashes to guide that puppy mind of ours.

Stress and worry are some of the biggest culprits when it comes to IBS flare-ups. While we can't always control external stressors, we can learn how to manage them in ways that reduce their impact on our bodies. When you live with IBS, even small worries can seem to spiral out of control, triggering symptoms that just make everything worse. But the good news is, you can take practical steps to manage stress and worry—and, in turn, manage your IBS symptoms.

Understanding Stress and IBS

It's no secret that stress can be a major trigger for IBS. It can set off that familiar chain reaction: stress causes IBS symptoms, IBS symptoms cause more stress, and round and round we go. Stress itself isn't always the problem though—it's how we react to it that often makes the biggest difference. For years, I thought I was just a naturally stressed person, constantly thinking, "I can't cope!" or "I'm too stressed!" But in reality, a lot of what I was experiencing was internal. The way I framed each situation, how I allowed my thoughts to run wild—that was what led to stress.

As Susan Jeffers[1] says: *"The greatest weapon against stress is our ability to choose one thought over another."* Before this, I was habitually allowing stressful thoughts and anxiety to run around in my mind without the realisation that I actually have control over that. It takes time, yes, but you can take back control.

Managing stress means both learning how to react to stress more effectively and reducing stressors in our lives where we can. This starts with reframing how we see stress—not as an insurmountable obstacle but as an opportunity for growth and learning. When faced with stressful situations, ask yourself, "How can I grow from this?" or "What am I learning here?" Reframing stress in this way takes away some of its power and allows you to handle it more confidently.

***

---

1. Susan Jeffers (1938–2012) was an American psychologist and self-help author best known for her influential book *Feel the Fear and Do It Anyway*. Her work focuses on empowering people to overcome fear, embrace uncertainty, and build confidence in their personal and professional lives. Jeffers' teachings continue to inspire readers worldwide to take control of their lives by facing fears head-on.

Relaxation Techniques: Progressive Muscle Relaxation

You've already seen how breathing techniques like rhythmic breathing can calm your nervous system (see page 72), but there are other simple relaxation exercises you can use to reduce stress as well.

This is a technique I found especially helpful when stress left me feeling physically tense. I could feel it right away in my neck and shoulders—it was all tight and knotted up. The great thing about this exercise is that it's simple yet incredibly effective. You start from your toes, working your way up to your head, tensing and then releasing each muscle group as you go. By the time you reach the top, you've likely released a lot of the physical tension that stress builds up.

Why Progressive Muscle Relaxation Helps: PMR works because it uses a combination of tension and relaxation, allowing your body to naturally shift out of stress mode. By consciously feeling the difference between tension and relaxation, you start to recognise where you hold stress and, more importantly, how to let it go. This exercise is fantastic for calming down, improving sleep, and easing symptoms of stress and anxiety.

Here's How to Do It:

1. **Set the Scene:** Find a comfortable, quiet place where you can sit or lie down and relax. Close your eyes and take a few deep breaths, settling into the moment.

2. **Begin with Your Feet:** Start by focusing on your feet. Tighten the muscles here—curl your toes or point your feet—hold for about five seconds, and then let go. Pay close attention to the release, noticing how different it feels from the tension.

3. **Move Up Gradually:** From your feet, work your way up your body, muscle group by muscle group. This focus on the shift from tension to relaxation is what makes this technique so effective:

    - **Legs:** Tense your calves and then your thighs, holding briefly and then releasing. Feel that contrast as the tension leaves each area.

    - **Core:** Tense your stomach muscles, then your lower back, noticing how the muscles feel as you release them.

    - **Upper Body:** Move to your shoulders and upper back, where stress often lingers. Tighten these areas, hold, and then let them relax fully, feeling the weight lift.

    - **Arms and Hands:** Clench your fists, tighten your forearms, then release, taking a moment to sense the relaxation that follows.

    - **Face and Head:** Finally, focus on your face. Squeeze your eyes shut or clench your jaw, then let go, experiencing the calm that comes with fully relaxing.

4. **End with Whole-Body Relaxation:** Once you've moved through each area, take a few deep breaths, savouring the sensation of relaxation in your entire body. You'll likely feel lighter, as if a weight has lifted, and you'll be more connected to your body's natural response to stress release.

This technique is all about noticing the shift between tension and relaxation—that contrast is what makes PMR so powerful. For an added guide, this audio version from Anxiety Canada can walk you through the steps. (Audio at the bottom of the page on the website) Scan the QR code for the Progressive Muscle Relaxation Link.

Journaling: A Tool for Processing Worry

Journaling can be a powerful way to manage stress and anxiety. When your mind feels like a tornado, putting your thoughts on paper can bring clarity. It's not about crafting the perfect essay—just getting your thoughts out of your head and seeing them clearly on the page can provide a sense of relief.

Consider starting or ending your day by writing down what's on your mind. What's causing worry or stress? Once those thoughts are on paper, they may feel less overwhelming, and you might even discover solutions or a new perspective.

Incorporate journaling as a nightly "mental detox." Think of it as emptying your mind's pockets before bed—a way to let go of the day's baggage and make space for peace and rest. If the idea of journaling feels daunting, remember: there's no wrong way to do it. It's simply a space for your thoughts, worries, and reflections—allowing you to let go and prepare for the next day.

By writing down your worries, you're taking active responsibility for your mental state. This practice helps you confront and release stressors rather than letting them linger and grow. I make it a habit to journal in a more structured way at least once a week, but ideally, I try to do it 3 times a week or whenever I feel stressed out.

Journaling Guide: Clearing Your Mind

The most effective journaling technique I've found came from an inspiring video by *The School of Life*. This journaling approach focuses on three core areas: anxiety, being upset with someone, and excitement or ambition. I start by briefly answering the three main questions related to these areas first, and then I dig deeper using six targeted reflection questions for each area based on what stands out the most.

The School of Life Channel

If you're short on time, just answering the first three questions can still provide clarity and be incredibly helpful. While I've adapted the wording of my questions, the essence and structure remain closely inspired by the video. Scan the QR code to watch. This method has been transformative for me, and I hope it helps you as much as it has helped me.

Journaling Video

Set aside about 20 minutes, grab a notebook or pad of paper, and follow these steps.

1. Briefly answer the three main questions:

- What am I anxious about?
- Who am I upset with and why?
- What am I excited or ambitious about?

Remember, this isn't a formal essay—it's a personal exercise, so don't worry about full sentences. Jot down words or short phrases that capture your thoughts. Just let it flow naturally.

2. Once you've written down your initial thoughts, move on to the six reflection points to explore each area in more depth.

3. What Am I Anxious About?

Start by asking yourself what's currently making you anxious. Anxiety can often feel overwhelming because it's muddled and unclear. Writing down even the smallest anxieties can help bring clarity. You might not know exactly what's bothering you at first, but let the thoughts come naturally. After you've written them down, use the following questions to help unpack these feelings.

Six Questions to Explore Your Anxiety:

1. Retell the story of this anxious situation in great detail. What exactly do you imagine might go wrong?

2. If things did go wrong, what would that look like? Imagine and outline the worst-case scenario.

3. Even if the worst happened, what strengths or resources could help you manage and move forward?

4. How would the version of yourself you aspire to be approach this situation? What would a more composed, grounded you do?

5. Does this situation bring up any memories of similar experiences? If so, what helped you cope in those instances?

6. Think about past challenges like this one. How have you successfully navigated similar feelings or circumstances before? What strategies proved effective?

Who Am I Upset With, and Why?

Now, reflect on any lingering upset you feel toward others. These can be small frustrations or deeper hurts. We often suppress these emotions, but writing about them allows us to process and release the tension. Take some time to describe why you're upset, and then explore the situation further using these six questions.

Six Questions to Explore Being Upset:

1. What was the upsetting incident? Retell in great detail, as if you were describing it to a kind, patient friend.

2. What aspect of yourself feels most vulnerable or threatened because of what happened?

3. Could there be another perspective on why the other person acted this way? Is there a possible explanation for their behaviour that doesn't involve harmful intent?

4. What are you worried might happen if this situation remains unresolved?

5. Does this situation remind you of anything similar from your past? If so, can you spot a recurring theme or pattern?

6. Imagine a friend is in your position. What advice or guidance would you offer them to address this issue?

What Am I Excited or Ambitious About?

Finally, turn your attention to any excitement, ambition, or positive anticipation you're currently feeling. These emotions can be incredibly motivating, but we often ignore them in the hustle of daily life. Use this opportunity to focus on what's lighting you up inside, and explore your excitement with these six questions.

Six Questions to Explore Your Excitement:

1. How would you describe your excitement if you were sharing it with a supportive, interested friend?
2. Imagine reshaping your life to align with this excitement or ambition. What might that change look and feel like?
3. What does this sense of excitement reveal about potential gaps or unmet needs in your life right now?
4. If this feeling could speak, what insights would it share about your current circumstances?
5. If this feeling were guiding you, what specific changes or actions would it encourage you to take?
6. What would your life look like if other areas felt as fulfilling as this one? How would it change your overall experience?

The Importance of These Journaling Questions

This journaling exercise helps you bring clarity and order to your thoughts. By taking time to write about your anxieties, frustrations, and excitements, you begin to see patterns and themes emerge. The six questions for each area push you to dig deeper, allowing you to process your emotions fully and take control of how you respond to life's challenges.

Make journaling a regular practice, and you'll find that fears, resentments, and hopes become easier to manage. Over time, this clarity will help you live with a greater sense of calm and direction. And another benefit is that you will 100% sleep better I assure you!

***

Stress and the Body: Belly Breathing

Stress doesn't just linger in your mind; it hits your whole body, especially the digestive system. One of the best tools I've found to help ease this stress is belly breathing (or diaphragmatic breathing). Belly breathing invites you to breathe fully and deeply, using your diaphragm to send your body a message that it's time to relax. It's simple, but the effect on stress—and even on your gut—can be huge.

Why Belly Breathing Stands Out: Unlike other techniques, belly breathing keeps things natural. While box breathing and rhythmic breathing rely on patterns and counts (inhaling, holding, exhaling), belly breathing is all about letting your body sink into a natural rhythm. It's less about controlling the timing and more about engaging the belly, which activates the "rest and digest" response, calming the mind and digestive system together. This makes it especially useful if you're dealing with the kind of stress that feels like it's living in your gut. When I tried it, I was amazed at how quickly it helped my body settle down—it's as though my whole system was exhaling along with me.

Here's How to Practise Belly Breathing:

1. **Get Comfortable:** Find a quiet spot and sit or lie down where you won't be disturbed. The more comfortable you are, the easier this will be.

2. **Place Your Hands:** Rest one hand on your chest and the other on your belly. This helps you feel the difference between shallow and deep breaths.

3. **Inhale Deeply:** Breathe in through your nose, letting your belly rise with each inhale. Try to keep your chest as still as possible and let your breath drop low.

4. **Exhale Slowly:** Release the breath through your mouth, feeling your belly fall as you exhale. This can feel really grounding and calming.

5. **Focus on the Movement:** Let your attention rest on how your belly moves with each breath. If your mind wanders,

just gently guide it back to this sensation—it's part of the practice!

I found that just a few minutes of belly breathing made a difference, helping me relax more fully than I expected. Incorporating these stress management techniques into your daily life can make a world of difference. Stress may be part of life, but with techniques like this, you have a practical way to handle it—and even keep your IBS symptoms in check—one breath at a time.

For a bit more guidance, this QR code offers a great step-by-step audio guide to belly breathing.

Taking Responsibility and Ownership

In her book *Feel the Fear and Do It Anyway*, Susan Jeffers emphasises that taking responsibility for your stress and emotional responses is crucial. You see, taking ownership over your emotional responses empowers you to handle stress more effectively, making you less vulnerable to IBS flare-ups. So please recognise that you have a choice in how you respond to stress and worry. Even if a stressful event is beyond your control, how you think about it and what you choose to do next is always within your power. Remind yourself regularly: "I am in charge of my mind and my emotional state." Say it often to yourself like I do in difficult times.

Tip #11: Practise Stress Acceptance, Not Avoidance

Instead of trying to sidestep stress, lean into it with acceptance. Recognise that stress and challenging emotions are natural responses and part of being human. By acknowledging these feelings rather than resisting them, you'll build resilience and regain control over how they impact you. Stress loses its grip when we face it with openness, making room for growth and understanding. Accept each moment as it is, and trust that you're capable of handling whatever comes your way.

Small Actions for Big Change

You don't need to overhaul your life overnight. By taking small, actionable steps every day to reframe your thinking, practise self-compassion, and develop stress management techniques, you'll find that your resilience grows over time. Much like building muscles through consistent exercise, practising moments of calm, mindfulness, and reframing thoughts will gradually improve your emotional and mental resilience. Remember, progress is progress—each small step you take is leading you toward greater well-being and better IBS management.

Tip #12: Commit to Daily Relaxation Practise

Integrate stress-relief practices like rhythmic breathing or progressive muscle relaxation into your routine, even if just for five minutes. Consistent, small efforts can build a strong foundation for lasting calm and resilience.

***

Gut-Directed Hypnotherapy: A Powerful Tool for IBS

I first heard about gut-directed hypnotherapy from a friend who was also struggling with stomach issues. Along the way, I discovered self-directed hypnotherapy, and to my surprise, a lot of it was stuff I was already doing—just not always in a structured way. Things like breathing exercises, visualisation, and positive affirmations were part of my routine. The funny thing is if someone had told me from the start that this was "hypnotherapy," I probably would've dismissed it as nonsense. But once I dug into the research[2] [3] [4] [5] [6] [7], I realised there's a fair amount of evidence behind it. And that's why I'm sharing it with you now—especially if you've already tried the techniques in the previous chapters.

---

2. Frontiers. (2024). *Gut-directed hypnosis and hypnotherapy for irritable bowel syndrome: a mini-review.* Retrieved from https://www.frontiersin.org/articles/10.3389/fpsyt.2024.01016/full

3. Monash University. (2023). *IBS: Hypnotherapy part of the solution - Monash Lens.* Retrieved from https://lens.monash.edu/2023/10/23/ibs-hypnotherapy-research

4. Mindset Health. (2023). *Hypnotherapy for IBS: A Safe and Effective IBS Management Tool.* Retrieved from https://www.mindsethealth.com/hypnotherapy-for-ibs

5. Patient Info. (2024). *Hypnotherapy for IBS: the gut-brain axis.* Retrieved from https://www.patient.info/hypnotherapy-ibs-gut

6. Peters, S. L., et al. (2016). *Randomised clinical trial: The efficacy of gut-directed hypnotherapy is similar to that of the low FODMAP diet for the treatment of irritable bowel syndrome.* Alimentary Pharmacology & Therapeutics, 44(4), 447-459. Retrieved from https://doi.org/10.1111/apt.13706

7. The Calm and Happy Gut. (n.d.). *Effectiveness of gut-directed hypnotherapy.* Retrieved fromhttps://thecalmandhappygut.com/effectiveness-of-gut-directed-hypnotherapy

Gut-directed hypnotherapy has definitely become a go-to treatment for IBS these days, particularly as our understanding of the gut-brain axis has deepened. Usually, working with a trained therapist, this approach uses focused relaxation techniques and visualisations that help calm the gut by reducing stress and anxiety. The goal is simple: to improve communication between the gut and brain, reducing IBS symptoms by teaching the body how to better handle stress and discomfort.

But why hypnotherapy? Well, clinical trials have shown that gut-directed hypnotherapy can have a long-lasting positive effect on IBS symptoms, even in cases where traditional treatments haven't worked. Studies have found that about 70% of patients who try it experience significant relief, and most of them continue to feel better even up to six years later. In fact, people who've gone through hypnotherapy are more than twice as likely to enjoy lasting relief compared to those who haven't. It not only helps with symptoms like pain and bloating but also improves quality of life by reducing anxiety and stress.

Similarly to the other techniques in the book, hypnotherapy can actually retrain the communication between your brain and gut, calming the gut's heightened sensitivity to stress and other triggers. It taps into the two-way communication of the gut-brain axis, helping regulate how the gut reacts and reducing the frequency and intensity of symptoms. I think that adding this to your routine offers a holistic, long-term solution to your IBS.

What's involved? Ok so, a typical gut-directed hypnotherapy session lasts about 45-60 minutes, during which you'll be guided into a relaxed state where you visualise calming, healing scenarios focused on your digestive system. With each session, you develop a greater ability to manage your body's responses to triggers that usually cause stress or flare-ups.

As you know, the mind and gut are deeply interconnected, and your mental state plays a major role in how your gut behaves. By lowering stress and anxiety through hypnotherapy, you're calming the gut's overreactive response. Many readers may have already practised some of the relaxation techniques discussed in this book, like visualisation and rhythmic breathing, which are also foundational elements of gut-directed hypnotherapy.

If you're curious, there are great resources and directories available online to help you find a practitioner. Alternatively, you can do what I did and start with some of my favourite YouTube videos to give you an idea. I have listened to these videos hundreds of times and yes, they help a lot. They also have a lot of other useful videos on their channels.

Please see the QR codes below:

- **Gut-Directed Hypnotherapy for IBS** – A calming and helpful video that introduces gut-directed hypnotherapy techniques.

- **IBS Self Hypnosis Session for Symptom Relief** – Focuses on deep relaxation and calming the gut-brain connection.

- **Sleep Hypnosis for Anxiety, Digestion, and IBS** – A soothing video to promote relaxation and gut health.

Self-Directed Hypnotherapy: A Tool You Can Use at Home

While working with a therapist for gut-directed hypnotherapy is highly effective, it can be challenging to access, especially on the NHS in the UK, where long wait times and high private costs can be barriers. Practising self-directed hypnotherapy at home allows you to maintain the results or even start your journey toward gut relief. Personally, I found this technique helpful once I'd listened to a few guided videos first. And the best part? Practising on your own is free!

How to Practise Self-Hypnosis: Self-hypnosis builds on the same techniques you learn in therapy, allowing you to manage your symptoms independently. Here's a step-by-step guide you can follow to enter a relaxed state and focus on soothing your gut:

Step 1: Create a Relaxing Environment – Find a quiet space and get comfortable. Take a minute or two to settle into the environment and ensure that you're relaxed and undisturbed. Listen to white noise or gentle nature sounds if you find it difficult to concentrate.

Step 2: Practise Deep Breathing – Start by breathing in slowly for 4 seconds and out for 6 seconds, releasing tension with each exhale. Continue this for **2-3 minutes**, focusing on the rhythm of your breath and feeling your body start to relax.

Step 3: Body Scanning – Once you've begun deep breathing, start a mental scan of your body from your toes upward. Spend about **3-5 minutes** scanning each part of your body, noticing any areas of tension or discomfort, especially around your gut. With each exhale, consciously release that tension, imagining it melting away.

Step 4: Visualise the Gut – After body scanning, focus on your gut. Spend **2-3 minutes** visualising your gut as calm, relaxed, and free of any pain or discomfort. You might picture a peaceful scene, like a river gently flowing, to symbolise smooth digestion.

Step 5: Repeat Positive Affirmations – In this relaxed state, spend another **1-2 minutes** repeating affirmations such as, "My gut is calm. I am in control of my digestion," to reinforce the calming connection between your mind and gut. You can choose other positive affirmations from the list below.

Step 6: Gradually Return to Full Awareness – Slowly count from 1 to 5, gradually bringing yourself back to full awareness. This step should take about **1 minute**.

Optional extra affirmations to use

Here are some additional affirmations you can offer for Step 5, which focus on calming the gut, reducing anxiety, and fostering a sense of control over digestion. They are all highly recommended ones based on research and popular wellness sources:

1. My body knows how to heal, and I trust the process.
2. I am at peace with my gut, and my digestion is calm and balanced.
3. I release all tension from my gut, allowing smooth and effortless digestion.
4. With each breath, my body becomes calmer, and my gut relaxes more and more.
5. I am in control of my digestion, and my body responds to my calm mind.
6. Each day, my gut feels more settled and at ease.
7. I am free from discomfort, and my gut supports me in health and wellness.

8. My gut and mind work in perfect harmony, creating balance in my digestion.

9. I trust my gut and allow it to function smoothly and healthily.

10. I am calm, relaxed, and free of stress, and my gut follows this state of calmness.

These affirmations are really about reinforcing that mind-body connection, promoting relaxation and a sense of control over gut-related discomfort. You can choose a few that feel right for you, or even better, create your own personalised affirmations that match your specific needs.

Practising regularly—just 10-15 minutes a day—can help maintain the benefits of hypnotherapy and provide a sense of control when stress arises. While sessions with a professional can offer more guidance, many people experience relief with self-directed techniques and resources like the guided videos mentioned above, as well as apps like *Nerva* and *The Calm Gut*, which provide structured support. (Details are below)

Gut-Directed Hypnotherapy Apps

Nerva

Nerva is a comprehensive, science-backed hypnotherapy app tailored specifically to IBS sufferers. Developed by experts in gut health from Monash University, Nerva offers a structured 6-week program that includes daily hypnotherapy sessions, education, and progress tracking to help users reduce IBS symptoms and manage stress. The price is £149 per year. You can get affiliate links where you can get at least 10% off. Nerva is very expensive in my opinion, but you could try the 7 day free trial and if you have the means to invest in this then I don't see why not.

The Calm Gut

This is a more affordable and flexible approach to gut-directed hypnotherapy, **The Calm Gut** app offers a solid introduction to managing IBS symptoms. It has a monthly subscription option (£11. 99) and a more affordable yearly plan (£119.99), it provides guided hypnotherapy sessions designed to calm the gut-brain connection and alleviate symptoms like bloating and discomfort. The app focuses on audio sessions that use relaxation, visualisation, and positive affirmations to help users manage stress and anxiety—key triggers for IBS. If you're just beginning your hypnotherapy journey, The Calm Gut's user-friendly interface and 7-day free trial make it an accessible entry point.

Final thoughts?

If I had the budget, I would probably go with the Nerva app for its structured approach to managing IBS through gut-directed hypnotherapy. However, the YouTube videos by Mark Bowden (a clinical hypnotherapist) have been extremely effective for me.

He also has his own app, Healing Mind, which looks great for those who want to address both sleep and stress-related issues along with hypnotherapy for personal development. Unlike Nerva, it isn't solely focused on IBS though, but it offers a 7-day free trial and some free videos, with a subscription cost of £13.99 per month. So it's still worth looking at.

I've also been listening to Michael Sealy for around 10 years, and his videos have been another great tool in managing my symptoms. So, while apps can be very effective, they're not absolutely necessary. There are plenty of free hypnotherapy videos online, and although you might occasionally encounter ads, YouTube Premium costs £12.99 per month (or £7.99 per month for students), which might be a more cost-effective option if you want ad-free access to all these helpful videos. In my mind, it makes sense to subscribe to YouTube Premium and enjoy these videos ad-free for less. I've also heard there are ways to watch YouTube completely ad-free using certain hacks, but I'll leave it up to your discretion to explore those options.

Reflection and Practical Step

Exploring Stress and IBS

Now that you've explored the relationship between stress and IBS, it's time to look at practical exercises that help you identify and manage your stress triggers. By setting aside time to reflect on stressful experiences and trying out the exercises discussed in this chapter, you can develop strategies to reduce the impact of stress on your IBS symptoms.

Exercise: Journaling and Reflection on Stress Management

Prompt: Try out the journal exercises provided in this chapter. Set aside 15-20 minutes one day a week to reflect on a particularly stressful experience. As you write, focus on the exercises that guide you through identifying your stressors and how they affect your body, mind, and IBS symptoms. Use the three main reflection questions from the section, and then work through the extra six questions to explore each area more deeply.

Practical Step: Mind-Body Stress Reduction Techniques

Now that you've explored different stress-management techniques, choose one to try out this week. These practices can help reduce both your mental and physical tension, making it easier to manage your IBS symptoms when stress builds up.

1. **Progressive Muscle Relaxation (PMR)**
   Try using PMR once this week, especially during times of stress or before bed. By focusing on relaxing each part of your body, you can release tension and calm your nervous system, helping your body unwind after a stressful day.

2. **Belly Breathing**
   Incorporate belly breathing into your routine, especially during moments of anxiety or stress. Taking 5-10 minutes

to practise can help activate your body's relaxation response and calm both your mind and gut.

Practical Steps: "Armour Your Mind" Against Stress

Next time you're in a challenging situation, try the following techniques to help manage your emotional response:

1. **Reframe Stressful Situations**
   Ask yourself: "How can I respond to this differently?" or "What is within my control right now?" Shifting your perspective helps you feel confident and in control rather than overwhelmed.

2. **Set Emotional Boundaries**
   Don't let others' negativity invade your peace. Visualise an emotional barrier—a glass wall or protective bubble—that keeps negative energy from overwhelming you while letting you engage with others.

3. **Develop Self-Compassion**
   When faced with stress, replace self-criticism with kindness. Acknowledge that you're doing your best and treat yourself with the same compassion you'd show a friend. This mental shield helps you recover from stress without added judgement.

4. **Practise Mindfulness and Grounding Techniques**
   Stay present by using grounding exercises (like rhythmic breathing or observing your surroundings) to focus on your

senses. Mindfulness, page 37, helps centre you in moments of stress and brings calm to your mind.

5. **The "STOP" Method**

   When stress builds up, use the STOP method:

   S: Stop what you're doing.

   T: Take a deep breath.

   O: Observe your emotions and physical sensations without judgement.

   P: Proceed mindfully, choosing how to respond rather than react.

6. **Practise Emotional Regulation**

   Recognise rising stress without reacting impulsively. Acknowledge how you feel, and choose a calming technique like rhythmic breathing or grounding to regain control. This helps prevent stress from snowballing.

By implementing these strategies, you can "armour your mind" against stress, building a protective layer around your well-being. This will help you face challenges with greater ease, just like the king who learned to walk across the burning sands.

Chapter 5

Emotional Triggers

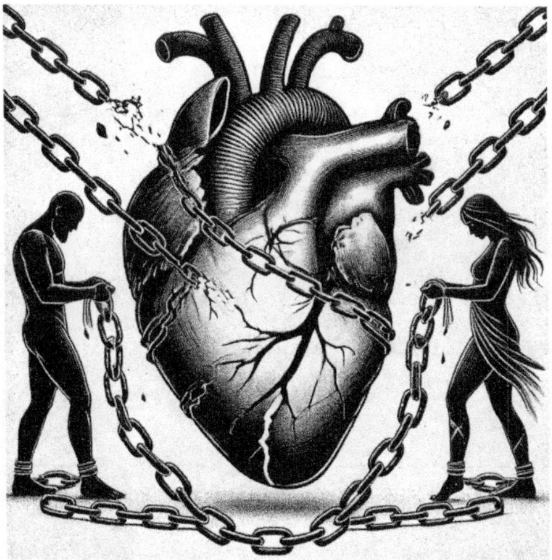

Emotions have a way of sneaking up on us, especially when we least expect them. For those of us with IBS, they don't just come and go without consequence; instead, emotions leave real, physical imprints on our bodies.

To be honest, talking seriously about emotions is a challenge for me. I've always leaned on humour and sarcasm as a way to avoid going too deep, often throwing in an inappropriate joke just to keep things light. But over time, I've come to realise that stress, pain, and unresolved feelings don't just vanish. One thing I learned from Dr. Bessel van der Kolk[1] is that the body doesn't simply forget painful emotions or experiences. Instead, it stores them, holding onto trauma, stress, and unprocessed feelings that can, over time, lead to real physical symptoms. When we suppress these emotions, they don't go away—they build up, creating tension and strain that affect our overall health.

Growing up, I often received the message—subtly, almost as if through osmosis—that showing emotions, especially sadness or tears, wasn't okay. Even now, if I feel that familiar burn of tears coming, my automatic reaction is to hide. There's nothing wrong with wanting privacy, but constantly shutting down those feelings is another story.

In the past, I tried "managing" my emotions by suppressing them or, worse, drowning them out with a drink or two. Alcohol, I thought, would smooth over the sharp edges and let me move on. But numbing

---

1. Dr. Bessel van der Kolk, a psychiatrist and trauma specialist, explores how traumatic experiences are stored in the body in his influential book *The Body Keeps the Score*.

emotions this way only made the problem worse over time, especially with IBS. I found that suppressing feelings wasn't a solution; it was a way of deferring pain, adding layers of stress that intensified my symptoms instead of easing them.

This kind of emotional avoidance leads to a feedback loop: we push feelings away, hoping they'll dissolve on their own, but unprocessed emotions just sink deeper and deeper, settling into the dark edges of the mind and gut. The body, as I've learned, keeps score. If we don't give ourselves permission to feel, these emotions stay with us, building tension we can't escape.

In the pages ahead, we'll explore a different approach—one where we accept and process our emotions with curiosity and compassion, without trying to drown them out. This journey isn't about "getting over" or "fixing" feelings; it's about allowing ourselves to be fully present with whatever comes up. From there, we can start to free ourselves from the weight of carrying unprocessed emotions. Embracing, observing, and working with emotions won't just help you find emotional relief; it will create a foundation of resilience, bringing peace to both body and mind.

There's a wealth of insights here, each offering a unique perspective. I included them all because each approach has supported me in some way, and I wanted to give you the chance to find what resonates with you. My suggestion is to explore whichever ideas or methods feel most meaningful; let those be the paths you pursue. It's not about trying everything at once but finding the approaches that feel right for you, so you don't have to sift through endless perspectives like I did. Choose what feels valuable, and trust that it will support you on your journey.

***

Acknowledging and Accepting Emotions

I first found Pema Chödrön's[2] work during a dark chapter in my life. Her perspective on embracing pain, rather than hiding from it, became a lifeline. Instead of offering quick fixes, Pema invites us to sit with discomfort—to acknowledge it fully, without trying to push it away. For anyone, but especially for those of us dealing with something as physically impactful as IBS, her approach can feel both challenging and liberating.

In the next section, I'll share some of Pema's insights that have truly stuck with me and shaped how I navigate my own emotional landscape. Her teachings don't promise a way to escape pain but rather a way to change our relationship with it, especially when emotions like frustration, fear, or sadness can intensify physical symptoms. Pema

---

2. Pema Chödrön is an American-born Buddhist nun, teacher, and author known for her accessible teachings on mindfulness, compassion, and resilience. A senior teacher in the Shambhala Buddhist lineage, she shares practical wisdom for working with life's challenges.

encourages us to meet our feelings with compassion rather than criticism, reminding us that emotions don't need to be fixed—they simply need to be felt, observed, and then released.

Allowing Emotions to Be: Embracing Pain Rather Than Resisting It

Pema emphasises that we don't need to categorise emotions as "good" or "bad"; they're simply part of our experience. By allowing emotions to arise without judgement, we can reduce their intensity. She often uses the term "leaning into the sharp points" to describe this process—by staying present with what's uncomfortable, we build resilience.

- *Example for Reflection:* Think back to a moment of intense frustration. Instead of shoving it down, try saying, "This is frustration; I see it." This simple acknowledgement keeps the feeling from spiralling and gives it room to exist without taking over.

- *Practical Tip:* When you feel discomfort rising, take a deep breath and repeat a gentle mantra like, "This is temporary; I can be here with it."

Tip #13: Allow Emotions to Exist Without Judgment

Let your emotions come and go without labelling them as "good" or "bad." By simply acknowledging each feeling, you allow it to pass without intensifying it. Approach these moments with compassion, recognising that emotions are natural and temporary. This acceptance creates space for healing and resilience.

Meeting Discomfort with an Open Heart

Another of Pema's essential teachings is what she calls "unconditional friendliness." This practice means treating ourselves with the same kindness we'd offer to a close friend. When dealing with high-stress moments or physical symptoms, try approaching yourself with patience instead of frustration.

- *Example for Reflection:* On a rough day, when symptoms flare, and you feel drained, remind yourself, "It's okay; I'm doing the best I can." Practising self-kindness can turn these moments from struggles into opportunities for compassion.
- *Practical Tip:* Place a hand on your heart during tough moments and say, "I'm here with this; I'm doing my best." This small gesture reinforces self-acceptance, grounding you in the present.

Learning to Let Go

Pema also speaks to the power of "letting go" of painful moments once we've processed them. We often carry residual pain, letting it linger and affect us long after the situation has passed. Letting go doesn't mean ignoring pain—it's about feeling it fully, then releasing it so it doesn't continue to weigh us down.

- *Example for Reflection:* After a stressful event, rather than letting it stew, acknowledge it—"That was hard, but I'm letting it stay in the past." This small reminder helps prevent emotions from building up into long-term stress.
- *Practical Tip:* Use a small ritual, like taking a deep breath or repeating, "I'm moving forward," as a way to release lingering feelings. This shift can help reduce stress and the physical tension it brings.

Key Takeaways:

- Approach emotions without judgement.
- Build self-kindness to transform struggles into opportunities for growth.
- Let go of past stress, using rituals like deep breathing to stay grounded.

If you're interested in exploring more from Pema Chödrön, I especially recommend *When Things Fall Apart*, where she shares transformative insights on finding courage and compassion in difficult times. She has many other wonderful books that dive deeper into mindfulness and resilience, along with some excellent talks available on YouTube. I've also found *The Pema Chodron Audio Collection* on Audible particularly useful (scan QR code).

***

Radical Acceptance

The concept of *Radical Acceptance* originated in Dialectical Behaviour Therapy (DBT), developed by psychologist Marsha Linehan, and has since been popularised by figures like Tara Brach[3] . This approach teaches us to acknowledge reality exactly as it is. Brach explains that accepting emotions doesn't mean we condone or enjoy them; rather, we allow them to arise and exist without judgement. By shifting our

---

3. Tara Brach is a psychologist, meditation teacher, and author known for integrating Western psychology with Eastern spiritual practices. She is the author of *Radical Acceptance* and *Radical Compassion*, and her teachings emphasise mindfulness and self-compassion.

focus from trying to control every outcome to accepting what we can't change, *Radical Acceptance* frees us from the exhausting cycle of resistance.

Imagine you're stuck in traffic, running late to an important meeting. You're frustrated, mentally berating yourself for not leaving earlier or blaming the drivers around you. Radical Acceptance would mean pausing to acknowledge that the situation is beyond your control. You may not like it, but once you let go of trying to change the unchangeable, you can shift your focus toward constructive actions—like informing someone you'll be late and focusing on breathing to reduce stress.

To guide this process, Brach introduces a now very popular method she calls *RAIN*—Recognise, Allow, Investigate, and Nurture. This practice encourages us to step back, examine our feelings without judgement, and nurture ourselves through them. Rather than building defences, we become more aware of our inner experiences, allowing space for emotions to exist without defining us.

Quick Steps for RAIN:

1. **Recognise** what you're feeling (e.g., "I'm feeling anxious").
2. **Allow** the feeling to be there without trying to change it.
3. **Investigate** with curiosity, asking questions like, "Where do I feel this in my body?"

4. **Nurture** yourself with kindness—perhaps placing a hand on your heart or using a soothing phrase like, "It's okay to feel this way."

Practical Example (Using the RAIN Method)

Imagine you're preparing dinner, and you accidentally spill a pot of sauce you've been working on. Instantly, frustration and annoyance surge up as you see the mess and realise you'll need to start over.

1. **Recognise** – Notice the frustration and label it: "There is frustration here."

2. **Allow** – Give yourself permission to feel frustrated without immediately trying to brush it off. Let the feeling be present for a moment.

3. **Investigate** – Ask yourself where you feel this frustration in your body. Maybe it's a clenching in your fists or a flutter of heat in your chest. Notice any thoughts fueling the feeling, like "I should have been more careful" or "Now I've wasted time."

4. **Nurture** – Offer yourself a comforting phrase, such as, "It's okay; mistakes happen," or try placing a hand on your heart as a gentle gesture.

By working through RAIN, you shift from feeling engulfed by frustration to observing it with compassion. This simple pause can help ease the tension, allowing you to clean up calmly and focus on preparing the meal again, free from lingering irritation.

In my own life, I've always been a bit of a control freak—an over-preparer, meticulous, and a perfectionist. I felt that if I could manage every detail, things would go smoothly, and I wouldn't face disappointment. But there were times, especially when dealing with loved ones or my own limitations, when I simply couldn't change things, no matter how hard I tried. Learning to accept these situations, to allow them to be as they were, brought a surprising sense of peace. While the pain didn't disappear, my perspective shifted, helping me avoid the exhausting cycle of fighting against reality.

Key Takeaways:

- Radical Acceptance allows for realistic, non-judgmental acknowledgement of emotions.
- The RAIN method helps manage strong feelings without defensiveness.
- Kindness and nurturing create inner stability, reducing stress impact.

Practising Acceptance

Here's a set of simple practices inspired by Pema Chödrön and Tara Brach to help you start acknowledging and allowing emotions:

- **Notice Resistance**: Watch for phrases like "should," "if only," or "why me?" These are often signs of resistance. Just noticing this tendency can be a first step in letting go.

- **Pause and Breathe**: When you feel an emotion rise, stop for a moment and take a slow breath. Imagine this breath as an invitation to experience the feeling rather than push it away.

- **Name the Emotion**: Try saying, "This is sadness," or "This is fear." Naming the emotion creates a sense of distance, allowing you to see it clearly without becoming engulfed.

- **Set a Time for Release**: If an emotion feels intense, give yourself permission to fully feel it for a set time. Afterwards, remind yourself that it doesn't have to stay forever.

Pema Chödrön and Tara Brach teach that emotions, when acknowledged without judgement, lose much of their power over us. The goal isn't to get rid of emotions but to change how we relate to them, transforming our internal landscape. By practising acceptance, we begin to reduce the grip that difficult emotions have on our physical and emotional health, creating more room for peace and resilience in the process.

Observing Emotions Without Attachment

Once we've started to accept our emotions, the next challenge is learning to observe them without getting swept away. Emotions, especially intense ones, can feel like tidal waves, rising up and crashing over us, colouring everything we experience. But what if we could learn to view emotions with a gentle detachment—not pushing them away, but allowing them to flow through us naturally, like waves on the ocean? For those of us with IBS, learning to let emotions pass can be particularly powerful, as the effects of stress and intense feelings don't just linger in our minds; they often settle into our bodies as well.

This practice of observing emotions without attachment is rooted in Zen teachings and mindfulness practices. Rather than labelling emotions as "good" or "bad," or holding onto them long after they've come and gone, we can learn to let each one rise and fall like passing weather. By cultivating this approach, we experience emotions fully, allowing them to drift away rather than letting them take over. Embracing this mindset can be liberating and physically relieving, offering us a way to move through life with greater ease and balance, even when emotions run high.

The Art of Letting Go

One of my favourite Zen parables beautifully illustrates the power of letting go. I've come across it many times in different places, but here's how it goes: Two Zen monks were travelling together along a muddy road when they came upon a woman standing anxiously by a fast-moving river, clearly in distress. She needed to cross, but the current was too strong, and she looked helplessly at the river in front of her, unsure of what to do. The monks had taken vows of strict discipline, a commitment that included refraining from physical contact with women. For these monks, detachment was key; maintaining boundaries was central to their training and their spiritual path.

Without a word, the older monk stepped forward. With a calm determination, he picked up the woman, wading through the strong current with her in his arms until they reached the other side. She thanked him, and he nodded in acknowledgement before continuing down the path without a second thought. The two monks walked on in silence, side by side, the woman left behind, watching them disappear down the road.

As they walked, though, the younger monk's silence grew heavy. His agitation simmered beneath the surface. An hour passed, then two, yet he held back his frustration. Finally, he couldn't contain himself any longer. He turned to his companion and blurted, "Why did you carry that woman? You know we're not supposed to do that."

The older monk, looking as calm and steady as when he had lifted the woman, turned to him with a gentle smile. "I set her down hours ago," he said. "Why are you still carrying her?"

This story offers a powerful lesson: we often hold onto things—resentment, frustration, regret—long after they've passed. Like the younger monk, we can carry emotions or thoughts that weigh us down, replaying situations in our minds, stewing over them, rather than letting them go. Instead of allowing these emotions to flow naturally, we keep "carrying" them, letting them create tension within us. Letting go doesn't mean ignoring or suppressing feelings; it means acknowledging them and then setting them down, rather than letting them control our inner peace long after the moment has passed.

How to let go?

Well, what I learned from spiritual teachers like Eckhart Tolle was to create distance from the emotion or feeling. He encourages us to "watch" our emotions as if they were passing clouds, acknowledging them without attaching to them. Instead of thinking, "I am angry," he suggests saying, "There is anger within me." This subtle shift creates that distance, allowing us to observe emotions without identifying with them.

In our lives, this practice can help with emotions that tend to linger, especially those tied to IBS triggers. By observing emotions as they come and go, we reduce their power over us, allowing them to pass naturally without becoming entrenched. When we're not wrapped up in the emotion, it loses its grip on us, and we gain a greater sense of calm and stability.

Tip #14: Let Go of What No Longer Serves You

After processing an emotion, practise letting it go. Whether it's frustration, guilt, or resentment, learn to set it down, much like the Zen parable of the two monks. This releases emotional burdens that can harm your health.

The Ocean Analogy

Jon Kabat-Zinn, often considered one of the founding fathers of mindfulness in the West, developed the *Mindfulness-Based Stress Reduction* (MBSR) program, launching his *Stress Reduction Clinic* in 1979. I still find his meditations and talks inspiring, and turn to them every now and then. One of the metaphors he uses that deeply resonates with me—and has been especially helpful—is his view of emotions as waves in the ocean. Each wave rises, peaks, and eventually falls. Rather than trying to control or stop the waves, we simply observe them rise and fall. This perspective encourages the kind of non-attachment we're aiming for, showing us that emotions, like waves, are natural, temporary phenomena we don't need to hold onto.

He emphasises that by observing emotions without trying to "fix" or prolong them, we prevent them from intensifying. This can be particularly useful when managing IBS, as our reactions to stress can often amplify physical symptoms. Kabat-Zinn also encourages approaching emotions with a "beginner's mind," or a sense of openness and curiosity. Rather than categorising emotions as familiar or predictable, we can observe each one as if experiencing it for the first time. This allows us to respond more thoughtfully and prevents us from falling into habitual emotional patterns.

Tip #15: See Emotions as Waves, Not Identity

Think of emotions as waves—rising and falling naturally. Rather than getting swept up, just observe each wave with curiosity. This simple shift helps you let emotions pass without amplifying stress, keeping you grounded and resilient.

Techniques for Observing Emotions

Here are some techniques inspired by Zen teachings, Tolle, and Kabat-Zinn, to help you practise observing emotions with non-attachment:

1. **Noting Emotions** – When a strong emotion arises, try labelling it. For example, instead of saying, "I am stressed," try saying, "There is stress here." This slight change in language creates distance, helping reduce the emotion's intensity and allowing you to observe it without becoming overwhelmed.

2. **Visualisation Exercise** – Imagine each emotion as a wave, rising, cresting, and then receding. Visualise it coming and going, reminding yourself that all emotions are temporary. This exercise reinforces the natural ebb and flow of emotions, helping to prevent them from taking hold.

3. **Grounding Techniques** – Pair this mindfulness practice with grounding exercises, such as deep breathing or a body scan. As you breathe or scan, focus on physical sensations, bringing yourself back to the present moment. This can be especially helpful for managing the physical responses that often accompany strong emotions.

4. **Practise Curiosity** – Engage with each emotion as if it were entirely new, asking questions like, "What does this feel like in my body?" or "How does this emotion change over time?" This "beginner's mind" approach allows you to observe emotions without judgement, creating more flexibility in how you manage intense feelings.

Observing emotions with non-attachment allows us to feel without being swept away. Instead of pushing emotions aside or becoming consumed by them, these techniques help us remain grounded, recognising that emotions are temporary waves that we can let rise and fall naturally. This practice not only reduces stress but also brings a renewed sense of resilience, offering a way to experience emotions fully while maintaining peace within.

Key Takeaways:

- **View Emotions as Passing Phenomena**: Embrace emotions as temporary waves, rising and falling like ocean tides, to let them pass without attachment.
- **Let Go Through Visualisation**: Visualise each emotion as something separate, like a wave or a leaf floating away, to ease its intensity.
- **Create Emotional Distance**: Instead of saying, "I am angry," say, "There is anger within me," which builds resilience by helping to detach from the feeling.
- **Cultivate a "Beginner's Mind"**: Approach each emotion with curiosity, as if you're experiencing it for the first time, to prevent being swept up in it.
- **Practise Grounding Techniques**: Pair emotional observation with grounding exercises like deep breathing or a body scan to stay anchored in the present.

If you want to go deeper into Kabat-Zinn's teachings, here's a *Mindfulness-Based Stress Reduction* playlist (scan QR code). The recordings may feel a bit dated, but the wisdom in them is timeless and incredibly useful for anyone looking to cultivate mindfulness and resilience.

Also, here's a recent short meditation video (scan QR code), offering a quick immersion into his teachings. If you're looking for something a bit longer, his classic 45-minute body scan meditation (scan QR code) is a foundational piece from his *Mindfulness-Based Stress Reduction* program and remains one of the most effective for stress relief and relaxation. Finally, if you like his teaching style and approach, you might also want to explore his insightful Master Class on mindfulness and meditation (scan QR code), which I found both profound and accessible.

Body Scan Meditation

5 minute Guided Meditation

Master-class link

Embracing Vulnerability and Self-Compassion

We've all had those moments when emotions catch us off guard. It's the heart racing with anxiety before a big presentation or the sinking sadness after a difficult conversation. If you're anything like me, your first reaction might be to ignore it, to just "power through" or "man up". But when I first stumbled upon the teachings of Brené Brown and Kristen Neff, it hit me how much I'd been denying myself the space to actually feel. They weren't just advocating for vulnerability or kindness in some abstract way—they were talking about how we approach ourselves in the toughest of times. And in a world that often tells us to "man up" or "keep it together," their advice was a refreshing call to let go of that false front and be real with ourselves.

- **The Power of Vulnerability**
  Embracing the Full Spectrum of Emotions
  Brené Brown's work shines a spotlight on vulnerability, but not as a flaw or weakness. In fact, she sees vulnerability as the birthplace of courage and connection. Think about it: how much easier is it to navigate life while building up walls around ourselves? But that closing off eventually weighs us down. Brown's message is simple yet powerful: by letting ourselves feel, especially the messy emotions like sadness or shame, we can move through them instead of getting stuck. For someone managing IBS, this perspective has a practical purpose—unprocessed emotions can manifest in the gut, compounding stress. Allowing yourself to feel is a way of

releasing that inner tension.

Vulnerability isn't about oversharing or wallowing. It's about taking a deep breath and saying, "This is where I'm at right now." It's the courage to admit that, yes, some days are harder than others, and that's okay. Brown's work challenges us to open up to this vulnerability, not just with others but within ourselves, embracing what we feel without covering it up with a façade.

- **Self-Compassion**
  Kindness as a Response to Pain
  Kristen Neff's concept of self-compassion is like learning to be our own best friend. Self-compassion asks us to meet our moments of struggle with kindness instead of criticism. How often, when emotions get intense, do we tell ourselves we're overreacting or being "too sensitive"? Neff's work reminds us that we don't have to add insult to injury. For those of us dealing with IBS, where emotions can lead to physical symptoms, responding to ourselves with compassion rather than judgement is more than just good advice—it's essential for our health.

Neff breaks self-compassion down into three parts: kindness, common humanity, and mindfulness. Kindness reminds us to treat ourselves gently; common humanity reassures us that we're not alone in our struggles; and mindfulness teaches us to observe emotions without drowning in them. It's like creating a safe harbour within ourselves. When we stop judging ourselves, we make room to actually understand what's going on, whether it's anxiety, anger, or sadness.

This approach softens the impact of intense emotions, allowing them to pass rather than stay bottled up.

Kristen Neff explains the three components of self-compassion in this wonderful short video (scan QR code).

I can remember a time when I faced a tough day—work stress, IBS flaring up, and that constant nagging feeling of not being able to "keep it together." My instinct was to have a go at myself, thinking, "Why can't I just handle this?" "How is everybody else able to cope and not me?". But I remembered Neff's self-compassion teachings and paused. Instead of judging, I let myself acknowledge how much I was going through. I took a moment, a breath, and reminded myself that it was okay to feel that way. Surprisingly, this small shift in perspective calmed both my mind and my symptoms. Practising self-compassion in moments like these has become a way of reminding myself that, yes, I'm human—and that's more than okay.

Practical Tips for Self-Compassion

Here are a few ways to embrace vulnerability and practise self-compassion:

- **Speak Kindly to Yourself** – When emotions rise, imagine talking to yourself as you would a close friend. If you're feeling overwhelmed, try saying, "This is tough, but I'm handling it as best I can."
- **Affirmations** – Write down or repeat different affirmations like, "I'm doing my best," or "It's okay to feel this way."

These reminders can break the cycle of self-criticism.

- **Create a Supportive Mantra** – Find a phrase that resonates with you, like, "I'm allowed to take my time with this," and repeat it during challenging moments. This can ground you in self-compassion, easing the urge to be overly critical.

Brown and Neff's teachings offer a roadmap for navigating intense emotions with gentleness. By embracing vulnerability and self-compassion, we build resilience against the effects of stress on both mind and body, offering a little more peace to our lives—even on the hard days.

Below are some guided practices from Kristin Neff to deepen self-compassion, mindfulness, and emotional resilience, helping you nurture a more supportive inner environment. Highly recommend!

1. Compassionate Body Scan - A Guided Meditation by Kristin Neff

2. Soften, Soothe, and Allow: A Guided Self-Compassion Meditation by Kristin Neff

3. Kristin Neff on Self-Compassion

And you may have already seen them, but Brené Brown's TED Talks remain incredibly powerful resources for exploring vulnerability and courage:

1. The Power of Vulnerability

2. Listening to Shame

If you'd like to go even further into her work, here are some of her most popular books:

- *Daring Greatly*: A guide on embracing vulnerability to build courage and connection.
- *The Gifts of Imperfection*: Practical steps for letting go of who we think we're supposed to be and embracing who we truly are.
- *Braving the Wilderness*: Insight into belonging, authenticity, and standing alone in a world that often encourages conformity.

Key Takeaways:

- Vulnerability is a strength that allows for authentic expression.
- Self-compassion fosters patience and self-kindness during emotional highs.
- Practical tools help build resilience by encouraging gentleness with oneself.

***

Prioritising Emotional Energy

Even if you are among the 12 million people who've already bought and read Mark Manson's book "The Subtle Art of Not Giving a F~", his straightforward advice on choosing where to spend our emotional energy is worth revisiting. I mean I read his book a few times but it's so easy to just put it down and not take action on the advice we are given. And that goes for all the books, videos and podcasts we listen to. Anyway, let's get to it. So when it comes to handling emotions, Manson's perspective is refreshingly simple: we don't need to pour our energy into everything that crosses our path. Instead, by intentionally choosing what matters, we free ourselves from carrying unnecessary burdens, conserving energy for what genuinely deserves our attention.

Choosing What Matters

Manson argues that one of the most liberating things we can do is focus on emotions and situations that genuinely impact our well-being. Not every grievance or passing frustration needs to weigh us down; by filtering our emotional investments, we can focus on what truly aligns with our values. For instance, instead of stressing over minor inconveniences or past hurts that can't be changed, we can reserve our energy for things that bring us fulfilment and growth. Choosing what matters gives us the freedom to release those burdens that only drain us.

Confronting Emotions with Honesty

Manson's philosophy is blunt but effective: be honest about what you're feeling and why. If you're angry, disappointed, or frustrated, ask yourself if this emotion is helping or hindering you. By confronting these feelings, you're taking a step back to decide if they genuinely deserve your time and energy. Maybe it's a fleeting irritation or something that, when examined, doesn't actually serve your well-being. Confronting emotions with honesty gives you the power to release what doesn't serve you, allowing more mental space for the things that do.

Filtering Your Emotions

1. **Emotional Filtering Technique**Manson's concept can be turned into a practical exercise: visualise each emotion you experience as it arises and ask yourself, "Is this worth holding onto?" Picture these emotions like leaves in a stream. As they float by, choose which ones you'd like to pick up and which can drift away. This technique empowers you to make conscious choices about where to invest emotional energy, keeping your mind uncluttered and focused on what genuinely matters.

2. **Journaling Prompts for Selective Engagement**Sometimes, putting our thoughts on paper can help clarify which emotions deserve attention and which don't. Here are a few journaling prompts to help guide this process:

    - "Does holding onto this feeling serve my well-being?"
    - "Is this emotion bringing value to my life, or is it holding me back?"
    - "What purpose does this feeling serve? Does it reflect my true priorities?"

Through this filtering process, you allow yourself to choose emotions that align with your values, strengthening your emotional resilience and conserving energy for the things that truly matter.

Deepening Emotional Resilience Through Practice

As we navigate the ups and downs of emotions, having tools like grounding, visualisation, and journaling can feel like an anchor in rough waters. But, as with any tool, they need to be applied with intention to create lasting change. Here's how we can make these practices more than just "techniques"—let's turn them into genuine, supportive habits for emotional resilience.

1. **Body Grounding with Purposeful Breathing**
   I know we've all learned by now that "rhythmic breathing" can calm the nerves, but when you add intention, breathing becomes something far more impactful. Next time an intense emotion hits, try this: start your rhythmic breathing technique (for me, it would be my 7/11 breathing) and quietly tell yourself on the out-breath, *"I am allowing this feeling to pass."* This isn't about pushing anything away but rather inviting yourself to let the emotion rise, then slowly release, creating a bit more space for peace in its place.

2. **Focused Visualisation to Let Go of What Lingers**
   Visualisation, when done purposefully, is powerful. Here you can picture your emotions as something passing—a leaf floating down a stream or a cloud drifting in the sky. As you focus, watch it move away with each breath. It's an active reminder that these feelings don't have to settle in or become part of your day. By observing them as separate, you can find a sense of relief and ease in letting go, even if only for a moment.

3. **Journaling as a Release Valve for Emotions**
There's something freeing about putting a feeling down on paper—it's like letting a bit of weight off your shoulders. I know we already went through a more comprehensive journaling technique but going through short simple prompts can be really powerful when trying to process how you're feeling. Try prompts like, "What am I ready to let go of?" or "What is this feeling trying to tell me?" This isn't about reliving emotions but rather giving them a safe space to exist and then leave. Over time, this simple act of writing down emotions can be a powerful way to release the weight of things you may not even know you're carrying.

Key Takeaways:

- Not all emotions or situations need to be addressed; choose what aligns with your values.
- Honest self-reflection clarifies what deserves your energy.
- Emotional filtering allows for clarity, helping prevent unnecessary emotional strain.

Conclusion: Building a Lasting Balance with Emotions

Learning to manage emotions is a journey, not a quick fix. Every time you sit with a feeling, take a deep breath or write down your thoughts, you're adding to a foundation of resilience that supports both mind and body. It's about knowing that these practices—breathing, letting go, and journaling—are always there for you, each one like a small step that helps shift the balance toward peace, even on tough days.

While there is a wealth of guidance and knowledge here, you don't have to take it all on at once. Choose the techniques that resonate most with you, whether it's exploring the RAIN method, practising different visualisation exercises, or learning to filter emotions. The goal isn't to master every technique, but rather to connect with those that feel right for you and incorporate them into your life gradually.

And remember, it's incredibly difficult to step back and create distance when you're in the thick of intense emotions—especially when anger or sadness feels all-consuming, and the thoughts and feelings seem inseparable from who you are. That's exactly why these practices are so essential. They allow you to create just a little space between yourself and the emotion, and with time, that space grows. It might not feel easy at first, but I promise that the more you practise, the more natural it becomes to observe emotions without being swept away.

As you continue, remember that each moment spent with these tools builds a relationship with yourself that isn't about avoiding emotions but about handling them in a way that makes life lighter and a little easier to live. Slowly but surely, you're building a more peaceful, resilient way of being.

Reflection and Practical Step

Understanding Emotions

Now that we've uncovered how deeply emotions can impact us physically, it's the perfect time to turn inward and explore your personal relationship with these stored feelings. By reflecting on how you handle—or perhaps avoid—emotions, you open a door to insights that could be transformative for your well-being. Embrace this journey with a practical approach inspired by this chapter's insights, and begin to release emotions that may be weighing on both mind and body, paving the way for genuine relief and resilience.

Reflection Prompts

Prompt 1: From Humor to Honesty

Reflect on a moment when you used humour or sarcasm to deflect a difficult emotion. What feelings were you avoiding? Write down what it would have felt like to face that emotion directly and how it might have impacted your response.

Prompt 2: Exploring Emotional Layers

Choose one unresolved emotion from your past—perhaps frustration, sadness, or regret. Explore what layers might lie beneath it. Is there a deeper fear or hope connected to this feeling? Write down what surfaces as you go deeper.

Prompt 3: Learning to Let Go

Think about a time you held onto an emotion—such as anger, guilt, or disappointment—long after the situation passed. Write about how holding onto it affected you, and consider what it might take to let go. Describe any small steps you could take toward releasing it now.

Practical Step: Acknowledging and Processing Emotions

1. **Emotion Check-in**: Set a timer for a short, 3-minute "emotional check-in" each day. When it goes off, pause whatever you're doing and focus on what you're feeling at that moment. Simply name each emotion without judgement or the need to change it—whether it's anger, frustration, joy, or calm. This practice creates a habit of self-awareness, helping you recognise feelings before they build up physically. Regular check-ins help build awareness and reduce the impact of hidden stressors on your body.

2. **Practise "RAIN"** (Recognise, Allow, Investigate, Nurture): When a strong emotion arises, go through the four RAIN steps:

    - **Recognise** the emotion.
    - **Allow** it to be there without pushing it away.
    - **Investigate** how it feels in your body and what thoughts accompany it.
    - **Nurture** yourself with a kind, supportive response, as if comforting a friend.

3. **Visualise Emotions as Waves**: During times of emotional intensity, take a moment to visualise each emotion as a wave in the ocean. Imagine it rising, peaking, and then falling away. This practice encourages non-attachment by showing

that emotions are temporary, much like the ebb and flow of waves.

4. **Weekly "Letting Go" Exercise:** At the end of each week, identify one stressful emotion you've been carrying and visualise letting it go. Close your eyes and imagine it leaving your body, like a cloud drifting away. Pair this with a deep breath as a symbolic release, helping reinforce a sense of emotional freedom and closure.

Chapter 6

The Power of Your Mind's Eye

Healing IBS Through Imagery

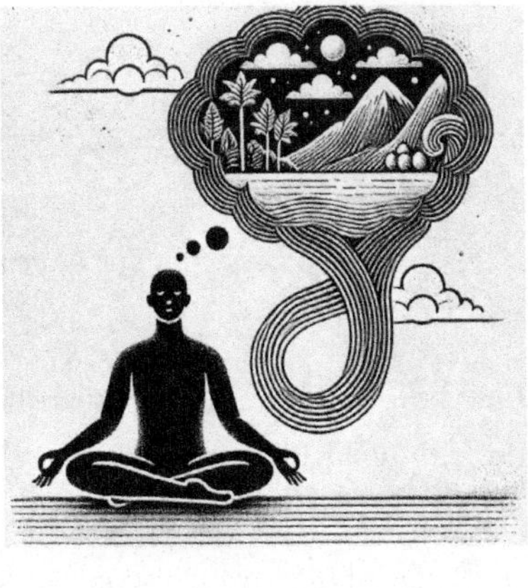

Visualisation is more than just daydreaming; it's an intentional practice where you use your mind's eye to focus on positive, calming imagery that can influence both your mental and physical well-being. When it comes to IBS, visualisation can be an invaluable tool in managing stress, reducing symptoms, and fostering a healthier relationship with your body.

It might seem strange—how can simply imagining things make a difference to how your body feels? But the truth is, visualisation taps into the deep connection between your mind and body, directly influencing how your body reacts to stress and discomfort.

***

The Science Behind Visualisation: Future History

> *"The mind makes it real [...] The body cannot live without the mind."*
>
> Morpheus (The Matrix, 1999)

As a twelve-year-old boy, *The Matrix* left a powerful impression on me. Watching it secretly at a friend's house on his VHS player (look it up if you haven't heard of it!), I remember being struck by its mind-bending ideas. The film stirred questions in me about reality, choice, fate, and most memorably, the remarkable power of the human mind. It was more than just sci-fi; it hinted at truths about how our perception shapes our experience.

The thing is, it's true—your brain can't distinguish between an imagined experience and a real one, which has powerful implications for managing stress and health. A famous Harvard study[1] highlighted this: one group physically practised piano exercises, while another group simply visualised practising. Remarkably, both groups showed nearly identical changes in the motor cortex of the brain, demonstrating that mental rehearsal alone can strengthen neural pathways almost as effectively as real practice.

In another study,[2] participants who visualised exercising saw an increase in muscle strength by as much as 13% compared to those who didn't practise any form of exercise—proving how deeply our minds can influence physical outcomes. The mind, in other words, "makes it real."

---

1. Pascual-Leone, A., Dang, N., Cohen, L. G., Brasil-Neto, J. P., Cammarota, A., & Hallett, M. (1995). Modulation of muscle responses evoked by transcranial magnetic stimulation during the acquisition of new fine motor skills. *Journal of Neurophysiology, 74*(3), 1037–1045. https://doi.org/10.1152/jn.1995.74.3.1037

2. Ranganathan, V. K., Siemionow, V., Liu, J. Z., Sahgal, V., & Yue, G. H. (2004). From mental power to muscle power—gaining strength by using the mind. *Neuropsychologia, 42*(7), 944–956. https://doi.org/10.1016/j.neuropsychologia.2003.11.018

For those with IBS, this connection is particularly significant. If you constantly visualise stress, worry, or discomfort, your body is likely to respond with heightened stress and more IBS symptoms. But by taking time to visualise calm, healing, and positivity, you encourage your brain to send relaxation signals, ultimately promoting symptom relief.

As with any practice, consistency is key. The more you engage in visualisation, the more your brain rewires itself to respond with calm rather than panic. Over time, this practice can make a significant difference in both your emotional and physical resilience.

***

Shifting from Stress to Calm

When I first started practising visualisation as an adult though, I still had my doubts. Could imagining a peaceful place really help ease the physical discomfort I was experiencing? But after a few weeks of regular practice, I began to notice subtle changes in how my body reacted to stress. My stomach didn't clench as tightly during stressful meetings, and my symptoms became less severe.

Here's how you can get started:

Step 1: Choose Your Visual Anchor

This is your mental "safe space"—a place or image that brings you a sense of peace and tranquillity. It could be a beach, a lush forest, or even a quiet corner of your home where you feel most relaxed. For me, it's always been the beach, with the soft rhythm of waves crashing in the background. You'll want to choose an image that you can easily recall and that immediately brings a sense of ease.

Step 2: Engage Your Senses

Once you have your visual anchor, bring it to life by engaging all of your senses. What does the air feel like on your skin? What sounds do you hear? Is there a particular smell in the air? Engaging your senses helps immerse you in the image, making it more real for your brain. For example, when I imagine my beach scene, I picture the soft grains of sand between my toes, the smell of salt in the air, and the gentle warmth of the sun on my face. The more detailed and vivid the image, the more effective the visualisation will be.

Step 3: Breathe into the Image

Now, it's time to connect your body to the visualisation. As you hold this calming image in your mind, begin to breathe slowly and deeply. Inhale for four seconds, hold the breath for four, and exhale for four. You can also try other rhythmic breathing ratios that we mentioned too. As you exhale, imagine any tension or discomfort leaving your body, floating away with each breath.

This rhythmic breathing helps reinforce the message of calm and safety to your body, triggering the parasympathetic nervous system (the "rest and digest" system) to take over.

Tip #16: Make Your Visual Anchor Personal

Choose a calming image or place that resonates deeply with you. The more meaningful and personal the visual anchor, the stronger its effect on reducing stress and promoting relaxation.

***

Visualisation: Reframing Stress with 'Future History'

Visualisation isn't just about picturing calm scenes though; it's about reshaping how you respond to stress and IBS symptoms. Instead of fearing a flare-up or worrying about how your body might react, visualisation allows you to mentally rehearse a different, more positive outcome. You create what's known as "future history"—mentally rehearsing an event in such detail that it feels like you've already experienced a successful outcome.

I've used this practice throughout my life. When I was younger, I was sceptical about its power, dismissing it as something my mother would talk about but never something I thought would actually work. However, when I was around 15, I decided to give it a real chance. I began using future history before every basketball game, visualising every pass, every play, and every successful shot. I even did the same before taking my driving test, sitting exams, and later on when giving presentations and workshops.

The shift was transformative. The more I visualised positive outcomes, the more my brain began to believe in them—and my body responded in kind. I went from being a sceptical kid to a true believer in the method. By mentally preparing myself in this way, I found that the stressful situations I once dreaded became much easier to navigate.

***

Practising Future History

When you practise future history, you're not just imagining a peaceful scene—you're visualising yourself navigating real-life situations with ease. The goal is to pre-create a successful "memory" in your mind, so when you're actually in that situation, it feels familiar and manageable.

For example, if you have an important meeting or social event coming up, spend a few minutes each day imagining the event going perfectly. Picture yourself feeling comfortable, confident, and in control, down to the small details—the conversations, the setting, and how relaxed your body feels. By practising this daily, you build a mental template for success, which your brain can access when the actual event occurs.

Tip #17: Practise Future History for Situational Confidence

Visualise upcoming situations where you might feel stress, imagining them unfolding positively and calmly. This "future history" method builds a mental blueprint for success, helping you feel prepared and reducing anticipatory stress.

How does this help with IBS?

That's all great, but how the hell is this relevant to IBS? Well, practising future history is particularly helpful for those with IBS because it reframes how you approach potentially triggering situations. By rehearsing positive outcomes, you lower the stress and worry that often exacerbate IBS symptoms. This mental rehearsal helps you associate stressful events with calm and control, which can contribute to a more relaxed physical response, supporting your gut health.

***

Healing Visualisation: Focusing on the Body

Another powerful way to use visualisation is to imagine your body healing and calming itself. When I was in the throes of my IBS symptoms, I would visualise my digestive system working smoothly, like a well-oiled machine. I imagined food moving gently through my intestines without disruption, the walls of my gut relaxing, and any inflammation slowly healing.

Here's a simple healing visualisation you can try:

1. Find a quiet, comfortable place to sit or lie down.
2. Close your eyes and imagine your gut as a peaceful, flowing river. The water is calm, clear, and smooth, flowing without any blockages or turbulence.
3. Picture any discomfort, bloating, or pain as debris in the river. As you breathe, imagine the current gently sweeping that debris away, leaving the river clean and free.
4. Stay with this image for a few minutes, breathing deeply and allowing your body to relax into the sensation of calm and ease.

Tip #18: Make Visualisation a Daily Practice

Visualisation can be your daily mental reset. Picture your gut as a calm, flowing river, washing away discomfort and stress. Just a few minutes a day—whether in the morning, during a break, or before bed—can make a real difference. Over time, this practice becomes second nature, helping you feel more in control, more relaxed, and ready to face whatever comes your way.

Visualisation in Action: Real-Life Scenarios

Incorporating visualisation into your daily routine doesn't need to take up much time. You can practise it first thing in the morning, during a break at work, or before bed. You can even use visualisation in the moment—when you feel the onset of anxiety or symptoms, take a few minutes to close your eyes, engage your senses, and breathe into your calming image.

Over time, you'll notice that this practice becomes second nature. Instead of allowing anxiety and stress to dictate how your body reacts, you'll have a mental tool to regain control and shift your focus back to calm.

Making Visualisation a Daily Practice

Like any new skill, visualisation gets easier and more effective with practice. Start small—maybe five minutes a day—and gradually increase the time you spend visualising. If possible, integrate it into your morning or nighttime routine. I preferred doing it in the morning because it kind of set me up for the day. The more consistently you practise, the more your brain will adapt, and the easier it will become to access that calm, peaceful state whenever you need it.

Cultivating a Healing Mindset

Visualisation is a powerful tool, but it's just one part of cultivating a positive health mindset. By learning to reframe stress, focus on healing, and practise mindfulness, you're giving your brain and body the message that you are in control. The more you visualise calm, positivity, and health, the more your brain will send those signals to your gut, helping you manage IBS from the inside out.

Even just five minutes a day can make a huge difference in how you handle stress and IBS. Here are some guided practices to get you started:

- **Headspace Guide to Visualisation** - This introduction to visualisation techniques from Headspace helps you practise focusing on positive imagery in simple steps. It comes with a mini 3-minute visualisation demo.

Headspace Visualisation QR code

- **Healing Visualisation Practice** - A 30-minute guided visualisation video. It's really effective for creating a positive mental image for healing.

Healing Visualisation Practice QR code

- **Beach Imagery Meditation** - Here is a 10-minute visualisation guided meditation with the image of a beach scene (my favourite) to visualise peace and tranquillity.

Beach Imagery Meditation QR code

- **Guided Visualisation Meditation** - Use this guided 17-minute session to practise visualising calm and healing with a gentle, supportive voice.

Guided Visualisation Meditation QR code

These resources can help you establish a foundation of calm that promotes both mental and physical well-being. So start practising now, and watch your body and mind begin to shift toward calm and healing. Just try one video and see what you think!

Reflection and Practical Step

Visualising and Managing Future Events

Now that you've explored the power of visualisation and how it can influence your experience of stress and IBS, it's time to put those techniques into practice. Visualisation, especially the future history method, allows you to mentally rehearse and prepare for upcoming events in a way that strengthens you, reducing anxiety and helping you feel in control.

Exercise: Visualisation and Reflection on Past Successes

Prompt 1: Visualisation of a Future Event
Think about an upcoming event that you're feeling anxious about—whether it's a meeting, social gathering, or a work presentation. Using the future history method described in this chapter, write out how you want the event to unfold. Be as detailed as possible about how you will manage your IBS symptoms, your mindset throughout the event, and the positive outcome you're aiming for. Then, use all those details in a 5-minute visualisation session. Go over the situation in great depth.

Prompt 2: Reflecting on Past Successes
Think about a time when you successfully managed stress or an IBS flare-up. Write about what you did, how you felt, and what techniques worked to help you stay calm or reduce your symptoms. Consider how you can apply these successful strategies to future challenges.

Practical Step: Combine Techniques for Stress Management

This week, practise not only visualisation but also integrate grounding or rhythmic breathing alongside it. For example, while visualising a future event using the future history method, start by practising a grounding exercise (like focusing on your senses) or using rhythmic breathing (such as 7/11 breathing). This combination of mental rehearsal and physical relaxation will help reinforce a calm, controlled mindset, ensuring you're prepared for the event both mentally and physically.

Part 2

The External World

Pause and Reflect

A Review of Part 1

Before we get going with the next section of the book, now is the perfect time to pause and reflect on the practices you've explored so far. IBS management is a journey, and it's easy to feel like there's too much to do or that you haven't done enough. I know how easy it is to passively read a self-help book, feel good for a day or two, and then move on to the next new book. That was my life for a long time. So, I know how it will turn out for you if you don't get started with trying all these techniques out.

The first steps are often the hardest—that's the nature of building momentum. Think of it as the snowball effect: at the start, gathering speed and building consistency may take effort, but once you start rolling, each action makes the next one easier. With time, the practices will come more naturally, and the results will start to compound, making a big difference.

And let's not get confused when it comes to consistency. It isn't about rigid discipline; it's about finding ways to keep showing up, no matter what. If you're low on time, try shrinking the task. When energy is low, go for a simpler version. It's not about sticking to a fixed routine but about adapting to what each day brings. Each step forward, however small, keeps you on track. Adaptability isn't the opposite of consistency—it's at the very heart of it.

It ***is*** difficult getting started, building habits, sticking to a plan, and being consistent—that's why I'm reminding you. So keep going, even if it feels tough. Ask yourself:

- Have I tried the breathing exercises or grounding techniques yet?
- Have I completed the journaling exercises, or did I skim through them?
- Did I experiment with visualisation or try reframing my negative automatic thoughts (NATs)?

Also, don't forget about two essential techniques we covered:

- Worry Time: Have you practised setting aside time specifically for your worries, allowing yourself to control when and how you engage with them?
- Rumination: Did you try limiting your rumination to just a couple of minutes, while using the three questions to shift

your thoughts toward positive or actionable reflections?

These techniques help lay the foundation for managing stress and anxiety, which will be crucial as we explore the external factors affecting your IBS in the upcoming chapters. As you move forward, here are a few questions to ground your progress and help you reflect on what you've gained so far:

- What practices have felt the most impactful so far?
- How might small, consistent actions make your journey easier in the long run? (Remember, it's about staying adaptable and showing up, even if it means adjusting the steps to fit the day).
- What's one small thing you can try today to build momentum?

These questions keep your focus on the small wins that, when combined, create the momentum you need to move forward. Take this opportunity to go back and experiment with the techniques you've read before moving forward. It's all part of the process, and there's no rush.

Chapter 7

Outside In

How External Stressors Fuel IBS

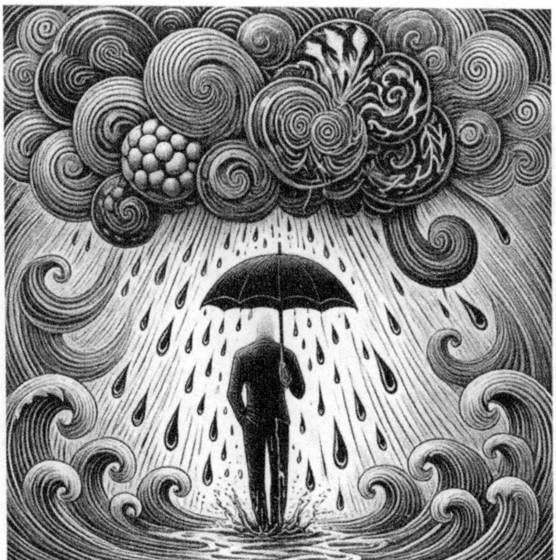

The Connection Between Internal and External Worlds

Up until now, we've covered the internal landscape—mindsets, emotions, and how they intertwine with IBS symptoms. But as you know, IBS doesn't exist in a vacuum. The external world, too, has its say in how you feel day-to-day. From the relationships you nurture (or endure) to work pressures, sleep patterns, food choices, and the lifestyle you lead, all these external factors can either exacerbate or ease IBS symptoms.

The connection between your internal and external worlds is like a delicate dance—one constantly influencing the other. You might have noticed, for instance, that even a slight tiff with a friend or a stressful commute can throw your whole digestive system into chaos. In this part of the book, we'll introduce the foundational concepts for external stress management before going deeper into specific stressors in later chapters. We'll break down these external stressors, explore how they contribute to IBS, and most importantly, discuss how you can regain control over these influences to foster a more IBS-friendly lifestyle.

***

The Web of External Stressors

Let's get real. While you can have all the breathing techniques, affirmations, and meditation practices in the world, external stressors will constantly test your calm. You might be thinking, "Yeah, but what can I do about my annoying coworker?" or "How do I navigate stressful family dinners that make me anxious?" These are valid concerns—and they play a huge role in your overall health and well-being.

It's important to look at these stressors in categories:

1. **Balancing External Demands:** Before tackling specific situations, the upcoming chapter, *Balancing External Stress, page 227,* will provide an overview of practical ways to handle various forms of stress that can impact your health. From workplace pressures and societal expectations to the hidden toll of perfectionism, you'll learn actionable techniques to minimise their impact on your gut health and overall well-being. Whether it's setting boundaries, refining time management, or shifting perfectionistic mindsets, this chapter offers tools to help you navigate external pressures with greater resilience and balance.

2. **Bonds and Boundaries**: Relationships are like mirrors—reflecting back both the good and the bad. A supportive partner or friend can be a sanctuary, while toxic relationships can act as major triggers for anxiety, stress, and yes, IBS flare-ups. Coming from someone who went through a very toxic relationship, I can confirm that the positive effect I ex-

perienced once I got away was like night and day on my body and general well-being. The impact on my mental health was profound, and, in turn, I noticed a clear improvement in my physical health and IBS symptoms.

So, in Chapter 9, page 245, we'll look into how your relationships—whether romantic, familial, or friendships—impact your gut health and emotional state. I'll also share more of my own story about navigating that toxic relationship and provide tips on fostering healthier dynamics that support both your mental and physical resilience.

3. **Managing Work Stress**: You know it, I know it—work can be stressful, whether you love what you do or not. Deadlines, high-pressure projects, and unbalanced work-life situations can be major stressors that contribute to IBS symptoms. I experienced this firsthand when dealing with a period of constant demands, difficult colleagues, and tight deadlines. The mounting pressure from work became a chronic source of stress that seriously impacted my health. Setting clear boundaries became essential, allowing me to regain control and reduce the physical toll that stress was taking on my body. This is why in Chapter 10, page 265, we'll explore practical strategies for balancing work and life, managing on-the-job stress, and protecting your health without compromising your career.

4. **Rest and Digest**: Lack of sleep or poor sleep quality can be like gasoline on the fire of IBS. Not many people realise

the extent to which sleep quality can affect gut health and overall well-being. A solid sleep routine is vital to managing IBS symptoms. In Chapter 11, page 302, we'll look at how to optimise your sleep to support gut health, discussing techniques to improve sleep quality and explaining why those extra hours of shut-eye matter.

5. **From Plate to Peace:** If you're like me, you've probably experimented with a variety of diets in search of relief. I went through the works—gluten-free, Mediterranean, fibre-focused, even anti-inflammatory diets—all claiming to be the solution for IBS. But after all that trial and error, the one I'd genuinely recommend is the Low-FODMAP diet. In Chapter 12, page 313, we'll dive into this practical, evidence-based approach to identify and eliminate trigger foods, then guide you on reintroducing them safely. We'll also explore how simple changes like mindful eating, understanding the gut microbiome, and even taking a second look at coffee and alcohol can make a real difference in your symptoms. The diet alone isn't the full answer, but when paired with other techniques in this book, you're on the path to lasting relief.

6. **Medication, Supplements, and the Role of Exercise Management**: Sometimes, diet and lifestyle changes aren't enough, and medication or supplements become necessary. I went through a journey of trial and error to find the right balance, and I know how challenging it can be. Some medications brought relief, while others had side effects that weren't worth the benefits. In Chapter 13, page 375, we'll

discuss how to assess whether a medication or supplement might be right for you, weighing benefits alongside potential side effects, and share insights into supplements that could support your gut health. It's all about finding what works best for your unique needs, with a focus on balance and long-term health.

7. The Long Game: Making short-term changes is one thing, but lasting relief from IBS has required a full lifestyle shift for me—and I can tell you, it's been worth every effort. In Chapter 14, page 407, we'll bring together everything you've learned so far, from mind-body techniques to dealing with stress triggers, and turn it into a sustainable approach to managing IBS.

When I first started, I was all about the quick fixes, hoping something would make an instant impact. But I eventually realised that it was the small, consistent actions—like sticking with the low-FODMAP diet, practising mindfulness regularly, and setting firm boundaries—that started adding up. It wasn't always easy or exciting, but over time, those little shifts led to a noticeable drop in my symptoms. My mental clarity improved, and I wasn't bracing myself for the next flare-up every day.

Long-term relief has come from building a routine that doesn't feel like work but instead supports my body and mind naturally. This chapter is about helping you find that same balance. With these tools woven into your life, IBS management can become a natural, even empowering part of your routine rather than a constant battle.

Tip #19: Commit to Action, Not Just Knowledge

It's easy to read about all these techniques and think, "That sounds great—I'll do it later," but later never comes. I know because I used to do the same thing. But reading isn't enough; it's the doing that counts. Real change happens when you take these ideas and actually put them into practice, even if it feels strange or difficult at first. Make a commitment to yourself to give these strategies a real try—start small, but start today. Remember, the only way to see results is to take action. Your gut will thank you for it.

***

Stepping into the External World

So this chapter sets the stage for understanding how your environment, external stressors, and lifestyle choices interact with IBS. The goal here is to help you connect the dots between the world outside of you and the world within you. Remember, it's not about changing everything overnight but about taking small, actionable steps to create a world around you that supports your well-being and IBS management.

Let's begin.

Chapter 8

Balancing External Demands

Stress Management Beyond the Self

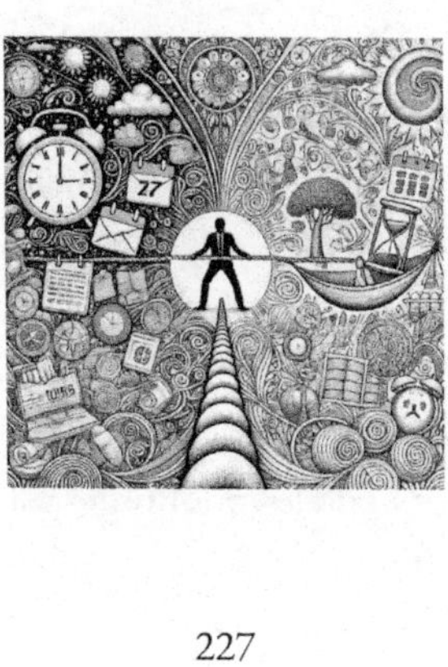

In Part 1, Chapter 4 (page 125) on Managing Internal Stress, we focused on internal factors—how our thoughts, emotions, and anxieties can trigger or worsen IBS symptoms. We explored techniques like reframing thoughts, practising self-compassion, and engaging in relaxation exercises to build internal resilience. While those tools are invaluable, we also live in a world filled with external pressures that affect our health just as much. Stress doesn't only come from within; it also comes from the workplace, social demands, and time pressures—factors we can't always control.

One of my childhood teachers once explained stress in a way that always stuck with me. She described it as a bucket that is constantly being filled with water. Life events, daily challenges, and emotional strains add to the water level. The problem arises when the bucket becomes too full—eventually, it will overflow, which, for someone with IBS, can translate into intense symptoms, flare-ups, and a sense of losing control. The secret, as my teacher emphasised, is to create intentional holes in the bucket. These represent the strategies and actions we take to release stress and prevent the bucket from overflowing. Whether it's mindfulness, deep breathing exercises, or engaging in activities that bring joy, these measures allow stress to flow out and maintain balance. But not all stress-relief methods are equally effective, and it's essential to be wise about the ones you choose to incorporate. Just as poorly chosen coping mechanisms may provide short-term relief, they could lead to bigger issues down the road.

Limiting the amount of water being poured into your bucket—essentially reducing exposure to external stressors—makes sense here, too. This involves setting boundaries, prioritising tasks, and being selective about commitments to ensure that your bucket isn't overwhelmed in the first place. By managing both the inflow and outflow of stress, you create a more sustainable way to keep balance and prevent an overflow.

So in this chapter, we'll shift focus to these external stressors—circumstances like workplace pressures, time constraints, social expectations, and more. These can make it challenging to maintain calm, which in turn, can exacerbate IBS symptoms. While removing these stressors entirely might not always be possible, managing your response to them can lead to significant improvements. From setting firm boundaries at work to adopting more effective time management habits, we'll explore practical ways to navigate these stressors without letting them take over your well-being.

Stress and worry are some of the biggest culprits when it comes to IBS flare-ups. While internal stress management helps us change our perception and emotional response, external stress management focuses on reducing or managing the sources of stress around us. Even small worries can seem to spiral out of control, triggering symptoms that just make everything worse. But the good news is, you can take practical steps to manage external stress and worry—and, in turn, manage your IBS symptoms more effectively.

Let's begin with an actionable step: identifying your main stressors. I know, easier said than done, right? But just as you wouldn't try to lift all the groceries in one trip (even if you've tried), don't feel like you need to tackle all your stress at once. Pick one manageable stressor and work on that. Small wins count. And each one brings you closer to the relief you're looking for. You're stronger than you think.

Start with what is most pressing or frequent in your daily life. By naming these stressors clearly—such as "work deadlines" or "commuting delays"—you can better understand how they impact your body and IBS symptoms. Let's look at some examples of external stressors that you may encounter and how to handle them.

Tip #20: Identify and Manage Your Stressors

Start by pinpointing the main stressors in your life. Don't try to tackle everything at once—focus on one manageable stressor, like work deadlines or commuting. Each small step you take to address a stressor builds resilience and brings you closer to the relief you're seeking. Remember, small wins add up.

***

Planning Ahead for Punctuality

If you're frequently rushing, the fear of being late can add unnecessary stress to your day and exacerbate IBS symptoms. Punctuality issues often come from feeling like time is out of control, which can make you feel anxious and flustered. These feelings, in turn, can worsen IBS. So, what can you do to mitigate this stress?

To plan ahead effectively:

- **Prepare the Night Before**: Lay out your clothes, pack your work bag, and prep your meals to save time in the morning. Small actions the night before can make a significant difference in how smoothly your morning goes.

- **Use a Planner or To-Do List**: Organise your day by writing down key tasks and appointments to keep yourself on track. A visual overview of your day helps reduce mental clutter and fosters calmness.

- **Build a Time Cushion**: Aim to leave earlier than necessary, allowing yourself a buffer to avoid the anxiety of rushing. For instance, plan to be out of the house 15 minutes earlier than your "latest possible time" to reduce the stress of last-minute delays.

Additionally, practise a morning grounding ritual—whether it's a short walk, deep breathing, or even a quick mindfulness exercise. These simple habits can help set a calmer tone for the day and reduce IBS triggers.

Tip #21: Prioritise Time Management to Reduce Stress

Use time-management techniques, like breaking tasks into small steps or trying the Pomodoro Technique (see below), to stay on track and avoid last-minute rushes. Consistent time management helps reduce the mental clutter that often leads to stress.

***

Setting Boundaries at Work

Work stress is often a major trigger for IBS, but setting boundaries can help protect your mental and physical health. Workplaces can be environments where boundaries easily blur, especially with emails, meetings, and deadlines adding to stress. By creating clear boundaries, you can establish a healthier work-life balance and better manage IBS flare-ups.

Consider these steps:

- **Communicate Clearly**: Talk openly with your manager or colleagues about your workload capacity. It can be uncomfortable, but setting expectations can lead to a healthier work-life balance.

- **Set Work Hours**: Establish a firm "cut-off" time for work activities. If after-hours emails or calls are a source of stress, let your team know that you'll be offline after a certain hour. For example, let coworkers know that you're available until 5 p.m. and stick to it.

- **Learn to Say No**: It's okay to refuse additional work or meetings if it compromises your health and well-being. Practise politely declining non-urgent tasks that overburden you.

Experiment with different phrases for setting boundaries, such as "I'm not available for this task at the moment, but I can contribute later" or "I'm currently focusing on priority projects, so I'm unable to take on extra work." Learning to say "no" gracefully can significantly decrease stress.

Work stress doesn't always disappear overnight, even with good boundaries. If setting boundaries doesn't reduce your stress, it might be worth considering a more supportive work environment or exploring a career change. Sometimes, a toxic work culture may not change even with boundaries, and seeking a new role or career path could be essential for your mental health. Be mindful of your body's signals when work becomes overwhelming, and prioritise your well-being over external expectations. **(Work stress and setting boundaries is explored in much greater depth in Chapter 9, page 245).**

Tip #22: Set Boundaries to Protect Your Health

Establish and maintain clear boundaries at work and in social situations. This might mean setting a "cut-off" time for work emails or learning to say no to commitments that overextend you. Boundaries create the space you need for balance and calm.

***

Taking Charge of Your Habits

Sometimes, we fall into routines like procrastination, overworking, or getting caught up in toxic relationships that seem impossible to change. These habits can slowly increase your external stress levels without you even realising it.

But even the smallest changes can go a long way:

- **Identify Key Stressors**: Whether it's time management, poor sleep habits, or work challenges, pinpoint the stressors affecting your IBS.
- **Make Incremental Changes**: Start small by adjusting one habit at a time—small improvements can lead to big changes in managing stress and IBS over time.

Recognise and celebrate each small change. For example, if you start waking up just 10 minutes earlier to give yourself a calm start to the day, acknowledge the positive impact this makes on your stress levels.

Remember, the aim is not perfection but progress. Small steps toward managing external stressors can significantly enhance your well-being and help in managing your IBS effectively.

***

Time Management: Easing the Overwhelm

There was a book I tried to read entitled *"Getting Things Done"* by David Allen. And I'll be honest—I couldn't finish it; I didn't have the time! But the truth is time management is another area that can create unnecessary stress. Procrastination and poor planning can make even the smallest tasks feel like mountains to climb. When you're managing IBS, the last thing you need is to rush around feeling overwhelmed because you left everything until the last minute.

So, trying out these really simple time management techniques can help ease the overwhelm:

1. **Prioritise Tasks**: Make a list of what really needs to be done, and tackle the most important tasks first. You'll feel more in control when you have a clear plan. In the past I wrote a list with different priority bands, and the ones on the bottom

just didn't get done. Also, sometimes just writing it out felt like a task in and of itself! So just write a simple list of things you need to do and cross them out one by one. It's that simple.

2. **Break Tasks Into Smaller Steps**: I'm sure you've heard it, "How do you eat an elephant? One bite at a time" If something feels too big or daunting, break it down into smaller, more manageable steps. Tackle one thing at a time. It's all about small consistent actions. Don't get caught up in the enormity of the task but instead focus on what you can do right now. Just like this book, at first I felt overwhelmed but I decided to focus on one small section at a time. And here we are! So, tackle one thing at a time, and remember—it's all about small consistent actions.

3. **Schedule Breaks**: Give yourself time to relax and reset. Scheduling small breaks throughout your day can prevent burnout and stress. One method I've found really effective is the Pomodoro Technique. This approach involves working in focused intervals—typically 25 minutes—followed by a 5-minute break. After four sessions (or "Pomodoros"), you take a longer break, around 15-30 minutes. Not only does this method help maintain focus and productivity, but it also ensures you're regularly recharging your mental energy. It makes even the most overwhelming tasks feel more manageable, allowing you to tackle your work one interval at a time. Trust me, those short breaks make a world of difference!

Take a few minutes each evening to assess how your time was spent. Celebrate what went well, and identify where adjustments can be made for the following day. This reflection practice builds self-awareness and sets you up for success.

***

Overcoming Perfectionism and IBS

Perfectionism can be a hidden stressor—one that sneaks into your daily thoughts, driving you to over-prepare, worry, and self-critique. Trust me, I know this firsthand. I'm a natural perfectionist and an over-preparer, and it took me years to recognise how these tendencies were contributing to my IBS. The constant need to "get things right" often leads to stress, which can trigger IBS symptoms.

Overcoming perfectionism starts with awareness and acceptance. It's okay to admit that you've been caught in the perfectionist loop; in fact, acknowledging that things won't always go as planned is the first step to healing. Once you realise that perfectionism is just another layer of stress that you can learn to manage, you're already making progress.

Recognising the Two Camps of Perfectionists

There are usually two types of perfectionists:

Over-Preparers

Those who find themselves diving into endless details, making sure every 'i' is dotted and every 't' is crossed, often at the expense of their peace of mind. If you tend to over-prepare, consider setting limits on your planning. Allow yourself to complete tasks within a set time-frame, and focus on finishing rather than perfecting. Ask yourself, "What's the minimum effective preparation I need for this task?" Once that's done, call it complete.

Avoiders

On the other hand, some perfectionists avoid starting tasks altogether, fearing they won't be able to do them perfectly. If this is you, focus on taking one small step at a time. Break down tasks into manageable parts and start with the easiest piece. Progress, however small, is better than staying stuck in place. Remember, starting imperfectly is still better than not starting at all.

Tips to Manage Perfectionism Managing perfectionism is about finding balance, and that can be done with some practical tips:

1. **Challenge All-or-Nothing Thinking:** Perfectionists often see things as either perfect or a failure. Start acknowledging the "grey areas"—a completed task doesn't have to be flawless to be valuable. Remind yourself that "good enough" can still mean progress and growth.

2. **Set Realistic Expectations:** Take a close look at your standards. Are they setting you up for stress? Allow room for mistakes and see them as opportunities for growth rather than setbacks. Not everything requires 100% effort, and not every task will have a perfect outcome—and that's okay.

3. **Prioritise Progress Over Perfection:** It's better to make steady progress than to hold back until things seem "perfect." Remember, done is better than perfect, and forward movement is what counts. Practise celebrating the small wins to keep up the momentum.

4. **Practise Self-Compassion:** Be kind to yourself when things don't go as planned. Self-critique can lead to anxiety and, in turn, worsen IBS. Speak to yourself as you would a friend—acknowledging effort, not just results. Ask, "Would I speak this way to someone I care about?"

5. **Create Boundaries for Over-Preparation:** If you find yourself over-preparing, set a time limit and stick to it. Let go of the idea that doing more always means better results. For example, if you're preparing a presentation, give yourself a set number of hours to prepare and then let it be. Your peace of mind is more important than that extra tweak.

Remember, Letting Go Lightens the Load

I've learned that letting go of perfectionism doesn't mean lowering your standards—it simply means allowing yourself to breathe. Perfectionism is a double-edged sword: it can drive you to do your best, but it can also make life unnecessarily stressful. Letting go, step by step, will help lighten the load on your mind and body. Remember, it's a journey. One small, imperfect step at a time.

Reflection and Practical Step

Managing Work Stress and Perfectionism

Work stress and perfectionism are two external stressors that can take a serious toll on both mind and body, especially for those managing IBS. Reflecting on how these factors shape your daily life—and committing to small, purposeful changes—can pave the way to a more balanced, less stressful routine. By setting boundaries at work and easing up on perfectionism, you're not only reducing the weight of these stressors but also taking back control over your health and well-being. Small shifts add up, helping you build a work-life dynamic that supports your journey to better health and balance.

Exercise: Reflection on External Stressors

Prompt 1: Identify Your Top External Stressor
Think about the one external stressor that most frequently affects your mood, focus, or IBS symptoms. Describe how it impacts you, and consider any small changes that could reduce its influence.

Prompt 2: Evaluate Your Work-Life Boundaries
Reflect on how well you set and maintain boundaries at work. Is there an area where you find yourself overextending? Write down one way to protect your time and well-being in this area.

Practical Steps:

- **Time Management with the Pomodoro Technique**Implement the Pomodoro Technique for one day: work in 25-minute intervals with a 5-minute break in between. After four sessions, take a longer 15-30 minute break. Track how this structure affects your focus, productivity, and stress by the day's end.
- **Redefining Success from Perfection to Progress**Choose one task today to approach with the goal of "good enough" instead of perfection. Set a time limit and stick to it, then

move on to the next task. Reflect on the outcome and any noticeable effects on your stress levels.

Reflection to Release Stress

Each evening, take 5 minutes to review your day. Reflect on what went well, where stress could have been avoided, and how you can make small adjustments for tomorrow. Writing down these reflections helps reinforce positive changes over time.

By reflecting on your work habits and perfectionism, and taking control of external stressors like work pressure, you'll create a more balanced environment. Keep experimenting with boundaries and progress over perfection, and see how these changes can make a positive impact on both your work life and IBS symptoms.

Chapter 9

Bonds and Boundaries

How Relationships Shape Your Gut Health

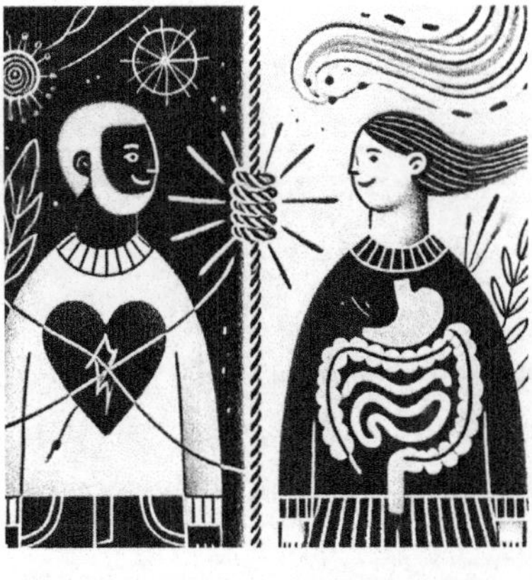

"The quality of your relationships determines the quality of your life."[1]

Esther Perel

When we talk about external factors affecting IBS, relationships come right to the forefront. The people we surround ourselves with—partners, friends, family, colleagues—greatly influence our mental and physical well-being. Positive, nurturing relationships can uplift, support, and ease the burden of stress, whereas toxic or strained relationships can cause emotional turmoil, triggering or worsening IBS symptoms.

Understanding the Role of Relationships

It's often easy to overlook the impact of our close relationships on our physical health, but connections play a pivotal role in either con-

1. Esther Perel is a renowned psychotherapist, author, and speaker known for her work in modern relationships, intimacy, and sexuality. With a focus on the complexities of human connection, her books, including *Mating in Captivity* and *The State of Affairs*, explore how individuals navigate love, desire, and trust. Through her writing, TED talks, and popular podcast *Where Should We Begin?*, Perel has become a leading voice in understanding relational dynamics and resilience in both romantic and personal connections.

tributing to stress or providing relief. Being mindful of how these connections affect you can be a powerful step in managing your IBS.

Think of it like an emotional "gut check": Do you feel supported, valued, and loved in your relationships, or do you find that certain interactions leave you feeling drained, stressed, or upset? Recognising the role that relationships play in your life can be a turning point in your health journey.

The Dual Nature of Relationships: Supportive vs. Toxic

The people around us can either be a great source of strength or, unfortunately, a source of anxiety. Let's break it down:

Supportive Relationships are built on trust, mutual respect, and care. They allow you to be yourself without feeling judged. Such connections can act as an emotional safety net, easing stress and providing support when times get tough. When surrounded by these kinds of relationships, it feels like you have an invisible blanket of comfort, shielding you from the weight of daily challenges. If you have people who uplift you and bring out your best self, nurture these relationships actively. Regular check-ins, acts of kindness, and open communication help strengthen these bonds.

Toxic Relationships are quite the opposite and can deeply affect your mental and physical health. These are the connections that might involve constant conflict, criticism, manipulation, or emotional unavailability. If you find yourself feeling constantly on edge, criticised, or belittled in a relationship, this may be contributing to your IBS stress. Esther Perel sums this up well: "We are wired for connection, but trauma rewires us for protection." When faced with toxic dynamics, our bodies can shift into "protection mode," where emotional tension takes a physical toll, showing up in symptoms like IBS flare-ups.

Tip #23: Prioritise Relationships That Energise You

Seek out connections that lift your spirits and provide positive energy. Surrounding yourself with supportive, understanding people can ease stress and promote gut health.

***

Toxic Relationships

While emotions like fear and frustration can flare up in any situation, some of the biggest emotional triggers come from the relationships in our lives. Our interactions with others—whether positive or negative—have a massive impact on our emotional state, and as a result, on our gut health.

We all know that some intimate relationships, friendships, or business relationships can be toxic. At the time, we might convince ourselves that we can't get out of them or that it's just something we have to live with. I'm writing this with a lot of experience in this area, and I'm telling you now, if you're in one of those difficult relationships, there is a way forward, there is a way out. Remember, on the other side of fear is courage and true freedom.

From 2013, I fell into a relationship that turned incredibly toxic, lasting over six years. I was in complete denial. Looking back now, I often wonder why I put up with it for so long. Truly messed up stuff happened—being locked out of my own house, sharp objects thrown at me, precious items smashed out of spite. Eventually, I gave up playing the guitar because every time I did something my partner didn't like, she would cut my strings. Friends and hobbies slowly disappeared, and I found myself utterly controlled—to the point of asking permission to leave my own house.

It's really embarrassing to type these words, you know. I thought I'd keep them a secret forever, but they're all true. I wish I could say all this made me stronger, but the truth is, I'm still picking up the pieces from that time. How did it happen? Why didn't I just leave? I don't really know. The abuse—physical and emotional—crept up so gradually that being hit, emotionally blackmailed, and made to feel worthless became my 'normal.' The bar for normalcy was just raised to a ridiculous point.

And I made excuses. To my family, my friends, and especially to myself. I thought things might get better if I gave it more time. But that stress was a huge factor in my IBS, even though I didn't make the connection then. I kept turning to IBS diet books and medication, never realising that one of the biggest problems was lying next to me every night. I was walking on eggshells, constantly trying to please my partner. The tension invaded every part of my life, including my health.

So, how did I eventually get out? Well, I found myself engaged (though I didn't even propose), and the wedding was looming. I remember being punished for something minor—maybe not wanting to go out or because of a private class I had—and my fiancée forced me to hand over about the equivalent of 500 pounds. That was the breaking point. I just thought, 'No. This isn't it.'

I ran like a scared rabbit, and of course, the fox came chasing after me. I ended up hiding in a dirty public toilet, and instinctively, I called my dad. Before that moment, I didn't want to ask for help—no one ever does, right? It's the shame, the guilt, the unwillingness to face how bad things really are. But as I perched on that porcelain prison, surrounded by shit-covered tissues scattered across the floor, a harsh realisation hit me: if I didn't act now, my life would be sealed in a direction I couldn't bear. I saw it—clear as day. Two kids, no social life, depression, isolation, endless arguments. It played out in my mind like a movie reel of everything I didn't want.

And that's when I knew I had to make my escape.

My dad picked up, and as I barely began to explain a fraction of what was happening, he cut in quickly: "Do you need me to come over there?" Normally, I'd dismiss the idea—"That's ridiculous," I'd think. "I can't ask my dad to fly 5,500 miles, spend all that money, take time off work… I'd be a failure, a laughing stock, the family embarrassment whispered about at gatherings." But this time, I didn't hesitate. I needed someone in my corner. I was just a shell of who I used to be, like a Dementor had sucked out the last circle of my soul.

"Yes," I quivered.

To make a long story a bit shorter—he came. He helped me through the transition, which, as he later confessed, was very difficult for him too. We broke up. I moved back to the UK for a while, losing everything in the process. I was still paying all the bills for our shared apartment until she finally moved out when the contract ended. It was a truly nightmarish time—but a nightmare doesn't even come close to what it really was.

Now I don't know you. I don't know what your life is like. But on the off chance that any one of you feels like they might be going through something similar, take some time to evaluate your relationships. Are they supportive, caring, and helpful? Or are they negative, dismissive, and cold? Think deeply about this. Your relationships should uplift you, not drain you. That heavy feeling you carry around in a toxic relationship can wreak havoc on your emotional and physical well-being, especially if you're dealing with IBS. Once I finally ended that relationship, I couldn't believe the relief I felt. Not just emotionally but physically too. It was as if the weight that had been sitting in my gut for years had finally been lifted.

So, if you find yourself in a similar situation, my mum said it the best: "Get help, tell someone, don't put up with it." Sometimes, family doesn't even know and might be convincing you to stay with him or her. Then, speak to people you trust and those who will listen. It really is crucial to reach out for support, whether from family, friends, or professional services. So, here are some resources available in English-speaking countries:

UK: National Domestic Abuse Helpline (for all genders): 0808 2000 247

USA: National Domestic Violence Hotline (for all genders): 1-800-799-7233 or text "START" to 88788

Canada:

- ShelterSafe (for all genders, with a focus on women and children): sheltersafe.ca
- National Domestic Violence Hotline (for all genders): 1-800-363-9010

Australia: 1800RESPECT (for all genders): 1800 737 732

New Zealand:

- Women's Refuge (for women): 0800 733 843
- Shine Helpline (for all genders): 0508 744 633 (24/7, also accessible via webchat)
- Aviva (for all genders): 0800 28 48 26 (24/7 support line)

South Africa:

- POWA (People Opposing Women Abuse) (for women): 011

642 4345

- National Shelter Movement Helpline (for all genders): 0800 001 005 (24/7 toll-free shelter helpline).
- Sonke Gender Justice – National GBV Helpline (for all genders): 0800 150 150.

Ireland:

- Women's Aid Ireland (for women): 1800 341 900
- Amen Support Services (for men experiencing domestic violence): 046 902 3718

Scotland: Scotland's Domestic Abuse and Forced Marriage Helpline (for all genders): 0800 027 1234

These organisations offer confidential advice, support, and practical help for those dealing with domestic violence or abusive relationships.

Remember, you're not alone, and there are people ready to support you.

Evaluate Your Relationships

Don't be afraid to end ties if you know they're detrimental to your mental and, ultimately, physical health. Toxic relationships—whether they're personal, professional, or even family—can keep you trapped in a cycle of fear, anger, and frustration. If you're in a toxic relationship, take a step back and remember that you have options. You're stronger than you think, and you always have the power to make decisions that prioritise your health.

Sometimes, it's easy to overlook how our relationships affect our well-being. Taking a moment to sit down and reflect on your personal connections can be incredibly enlightening. This kind of assessment not only helps you gain clarity on which relationships are supportive or draining, but it also empowers you to decide what changes you might need to make for your health. Whether it's setting boundaries, fostering deeper connections, or making the difficult decision to step away, reflection is the first step toward a healthier emotional space.

Depending on how much time and detail you'd like to put into evaluating your relationships, you have two options. For a quick check-in, use the journaling prompts below to gain insight into how your relationships affect your emotions, reciprocity, boundaries, and balance. If you're looking for a more detailed evaluation, check out the reflection in **Appendix A, page 461,** to explore these areas thoroughly and reflect on potential action steps.

Journaling Prompts

1. **The Impact on Emotions:**
    - List how you feel before, during, and after spending time with this person (e.g., energised, anxious, happy, drained).
2. **Reciprocity Check:**
    - Note specific ways this person supports you and how you support them. Is the relationship balanced?
3. **Boundaries Reflection:**
    - Have there been times you felt your boundaries were crossed? How did you handle it?
4. **Positives vs. Negatives:**
    - Write down a list of positive and negative interactions with this person over the past month.

Scoring & Reflection

After writing, score each relationship from 1-10 based on how supportive and healthy it feels. Then, reflect on what steps you might take to address or improve the relationship. Please refer to the Evaluating

Relationships Survey in **Appendix A, page 461,** for additional guidance.

Tip #24: Don't Be Afraid to Evaluate Your Relationships

Your relationships shape your emotional and physical health more than you might think. Take a step back and consider which connections lift you up and which drain you. Toxic relationships—whether with friends, family, or colleagues—can keep you stuck in a cycle of stress and exhaustion. You deserve connections that support your journey, not ones that pull you down. Don't be afraid to make changes that put your well-being first, whether it's setting boundaries or letting go of what no longer serves you. You're stronger than you think, and prioritising your health is always worth it.

***

The Decline of Deep Friendships and Its Impact on Well-being

It seems that as we grow older, friendships often slip down our list of priorities. Unfortunately, I've experienced this in my own life. Back in 2018, I came across *Lost Connections* by Johann Hari, and it really struck a chord. Hari points out that fewer people today report having a best friend, and many of us have seen our friendship groups shrink over time. Though we know this on some level, we may not fully grasp just how much loneliness and a lack of supportive friendships can weigh on our mental and physical health. These missing connections can fuel stress and anxiety, which in turn can trigger or worsen IBS symptoms.

Hari explains that over the past 50 years, people have gradually been spending less time together, leading to what he calls a "social crash." Studies have found that feeling lonely can spike cortisol—the body's stress hormone—to levels similar to experiencing a physical threat. This means that social isolation doesn't just affect our mood; it has a very real physiological impact. One surprising finding he shares is that many Americans now report having zero close friendships—a significant societal change that has contributed to increased feelings of loneliness and disconnection.

The effects of loneliness go beyond mental well-being; they ripple through our physical health too. A lack of strong social bonds can increase stress levels, disrupt sleep, and even aggravate IBS symptoms. Hari's message is clear: reconnecting with others, whether through social activities or even "social prescribing" (where doctors recommend joining group activities), can bring real improvements to mental and physical health.

Personally, I've found that joining groups and engaging in activities has been transformative for meeting new people and forming lasting friendships. For example, joining a guitar club not only connected me with others who shared a passion for music, but they also became my new family. Similarly, participating in a Tai Chi group gave me the opportunity to bond with others over shared practice and mindfulness. These experiences were great for nurturing friendships and had a positive impact on my stress levels and overall health.

If you're looking to expand your social circle, consider activities that genuinely interest you—whether it's music, sports, meditation, or something entirely different. And don't forget that volunteering can also be a great way to connect with others. It not only allows you to meet like-minded people but also gives a profound sense of purpose and fulfilment. Give it a go. If you don't like it then you don't have to go back but showing up is key! But you never know where those connections might lead!

***

Cultivating Healthy Friendships

Friendships offer more than just social engagement—they provide an emotional outlet, allowing us to share our struggles, express our feelings, and enjoy moments of joy. Taking time to nurture these connections is vital to fostering well-being. I learned this firsthand; I used to take my friendships for granted, rarely prioritising catch-ups or check-ins. But as I became more intentional about maintaining and growing my friendships, it had a positive impact on my stress levels and overall health.

When building or maintaining friendships, you're creating a space to connect, be yourself, and let down your guard. This can help lower stress and create moments of emotional release that are crucial for managing IBS.

Nurturing Existing Friendships

- **Regular Check-Ins**: Make it a habit to reach out regularly. Even a short message or call can show that you care.
- **Quality Time**: Carve out time to meet up, share meals, or do activities you both enjoy. It doesn't have to be grand; simple moments build deeper bonds.
- **Listen and Be Present**: Being a good friend is about showing up, listening actively, and supporting each other through the ups and downs.

- **Discover More About Your Friends**: Ask questions and be genuinely curious about what's happening in their lives. Often we stop inquiring as deeply into long-term friendships as we do when we meet someone new, so rekindle that curiosity.

Building New Friendships

- **Join Groups or Classes**: Find an activity you're passionate about—whether it's a book club, a sport, or a community class. Shared interests often form the basis of strong friendships.
- **Be Open and Approachable**: It might be uncomfortable to step outside your comfort zone, but be willing to start conversations and take the first step in building new connections.
- **Volunteer for a Cause You Care About**: Volunteering not only provides a way to meet people, but it also gives way to meet people, but it also gives a profound sense of purpose and satisfaction. The act of giving back is rewarding, and helping others can lead to increased happiness and reduced stress. Whether it's a charity, a local organisation, or a global cause, volunteering allows you to form bonds with like-minded individuals while positively impacting the world.
- **Be Patient and Consistent**: Friendships grow over time

and through shared experiences. Don't be discouraged if a new connection takes time to develop.

Tip #25: Focus on Quality Over Quantity in Social Connections

Prioritise meaningful, supportive relationships rather than trying to maintain a large social circle. Quality connections have a greater positive impact on mental and physical health.

Healthy, balanced relationships provide emotional support and peace of mind. They allow you to be yourself without fear of judgement, lifting the weight from your shoulders—and your gut. By recognising the dynamics in your relationships and making conscious changes, you take another step toward reducing stress, enhancing your emotional health, and managing your IBS effectively. Remember, it's all about taking intentional steps to surround yourself with the people who uplift and support you on your journey to better health.

Reflection and Practical Step

Evaluating Relationships and IBS

Your relationships shape so much of your daily life, from how you handle stress to how your body feels. If you've ever walked away from a conversation feeling lighter or, conversely, more weighed down, you know exactly what I mean. Taking a step back to truly reflect on your connections—and drawing boundaries where you need them—isn't just an emotional exercise; it's essential to creating a healthier, more supportive environment for yourself. By surrounding yourself with the right people and minimising emotional strain, you're laying down a foundation that lets both your mind and body feel at ease.

Exercise: Reflection on Relationships

> **Prompt 1: Evaluate Your Support Network**
> Reflect on the key relationships in your life—friends, family, colleagues. Do these relationships provide support, or do they contribute to stress? How do they impact your IBS symptoms, and how can you nurture the supportive ones while minimising the negative effects of others?

> **Prompt 2: Balance Connection and Solitude**
> Reflect on the balance between socialising and spending time alone. Do you feel recharged after spending time with others, or does it leave you feeling drained? How does this balance affect your IBS? Consider ways you can adjust your time to better support your well-being.

Practical Step:

1. **Evaluate Your Relationships**
   Go back and use the **relationship evaluation questionnaire** provided earlier in this chapter to assess the impact of your relationships on your stress and IBS symptoms. Take your time to honestly answer the questions and use this information to make any necessary changes in how you manage

these connections.

2. **Set Boundaries with Toxic Individuals**
   Identify a relationship that has been causing you stress. This week, set a clear boundary with that person—whether it's limiting contact or having an honest conversation about how you feel. Take note of how this impacts your emotional well-being and IBS symptoms.

By reflecting on your relationships and taking action to nurture the positive ones while distancing yourself from those that cause stress, you create a stronger support network to help manage your IBS symptoms more effectively.

Chapter 10

Managing Work Stress

Finding Balance in a Busy World

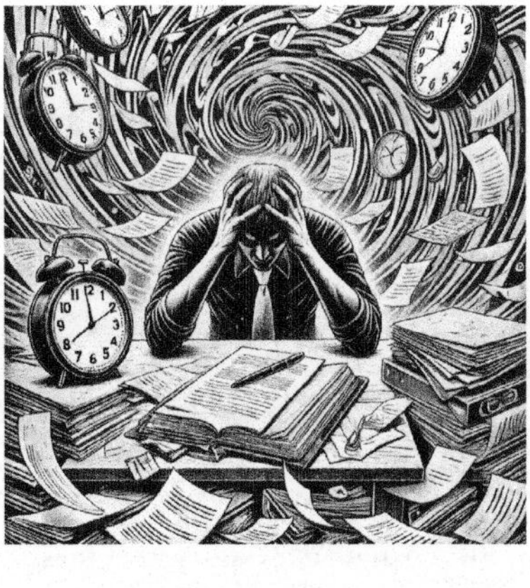

Before we get right into it, I want to give you a heads-up—this chapter is a bit longer than the others. But that's only fitting, considering how much space work occupies in our lives. We spend about a third of our lifetime working—that's roughly 90,000 hours on average! Given how deeply work intertwines with our daily experiences, stress, and overall well-being, it's only right that we unpack this subject in detail. There's a lot to cover, and rightly so, because the pressure, anxiety, and stressors tied to work are some of the biggest triggers for IBS symptoms. Let's get started then.

Everyone has work stress. I get it. The Sunday afternoon dread kicking in, a tightening in your chest as you mentally prepare for another bloody week. It's the constant internal politics of one-upmanship, power struggles, and the unspoken pressure to deliver—often all-consuming. At times, it feels like work-life has its own relentless pace, one that's impossible to keep up with, and the anxiety it produces can seem unbearable. I know this feeling all too well. At one point, I felt like I was swimming against the tide, struggling to stay afloat. I had full-blown burnout and had to take time off work. And even then I was worrying and stressing about things I'd be missing or would have to catch up on when I got back! My only option for overcoming this work stress was to leave my job, my profession, and even the country altogether! A bit extreme, I know, but I felt like it was the only way out. My body simply couldn't handle it anymore. My IBS flared, my mental health plummeted, and I genuinely worried about how long I could realistically last before, well, before I dropped dead!

So, how do we overcome work stress? Well, I found that it's not always about making drastic changes like I did; sometimes, it's the small daily habits that make a big difference. I think it's a mixture of managing workload, setting physical and mental boundaries, and getting the most out of your commute. But it also means learning to say no, developing techniques for self-care in a high-pressure environment, creating a supportive work network, and finding ways to bring moments of calm into the storm. All of this works together to not just manage the chaos but to help you thrive within it.

***

Understanding Work Stress

It's easy to feel like work stress is a dark cloud that's always just overhead, ready to rumble when deadlines loom, projects stack up, or office politics make every decision feel like a gamble. It shows up as that familiar tension—tightness in your chest, a pit in your stomach—echoing the pressure to perform and meet demands that sometimes feel relentless. At its core, work stress reflects the toll our jobs take on our mental, emotional, and physical well-being, an impact that runs deeper than we often realise.

One of the most challenging times during my career was a period where I had to give a presentation and lead a workshop to all teachers and staff. Public speaking was never my strong suit, and I dreaded the presentation for not even days but weeks leading up to it! My gut would immediately react—cramps, bloating, and that dreaded urgency to find a bathroom would hit every time I thought about standing in front of a crowd. I knew this wasn't sustainable, so I decided to change my approach. Instead of focusing on the worst-case scenario, I tried to visualise the presentation going smoothly by using the future history method (page 198). I also prepared by eating a light meal beforehand, making sure to avoid any potential triggers. For me, at the time, that was coffee! Slowly but surely, the symptoms became less severe, and I found that by controlling my mind, I could control my gut, even under pressure.

This experience showed me just how essential it is to manage work stress, especially with IBS. And while my stress was rooted in public speaking, work stress has plenty of forms, each impacting us in unique ways. Here are some of the most common culprits:

- **Deadlines & Workload:** Ever feel like you're racing against a clock with a mountain on your back? Juggling endless deadlines and responsibilities can turn your job into a non-stop pressure cooker.

- **Job Insecurity:** The fear of losing your job—especially in an uncertain economy—can feel like an invisible weight, a constant worry that's hard to shake off.

- **Conflicts with Colleagues:** Navigating workplace relationships can be like walking a tightrope. Whether it's a tough boss, an uncooperative co-worker, or a toxic team vibe, managing these dynamics can push your stress levels sky-high.

- **Unclear Roles & Expectations:** Ever feel like you're trying to play a game where the rules keep changing? Not knowing what's expected of you or feeling like your role shifts week to week can make work feel unpredictable and anxiety-inducing.

All these factors pile up, and when you're dealing with IBS, the toll they take on your mind and body can be even greater. Stress hormones like cortisol and adrenaline ramp up, activating the gut-brain axis, and IBS symptoms—like bloating, cramps, and pain—kick in. It's a vicious cycle; work stress fuels IBS, and IBS just adds more fuel to the stress.

***

Why Work Stress Hits Differently

Unlike other sources of stress that may come and go, work stress is **constant, daily, and often unavoidable.** Think about it—every Monday rolls around like clockwork, bringing with it the pressure to perform. The problem with work stress is the lack of control. You don't always have a say over your workload, the deadlines, or even the people you work with, which can make you feel like a passenger in your own life, instead of being in the driver's seat.

Work stress doesn't just affect your 9 to 5; it seeps into every aspect of your day. I would take my work home and if I didn't, I would be thinking about it every evening. I'd wake up with work on my mind, rush through the commute with a tight feeling in my chest, and replay the day's stressful moments when I'm supposed to be winding down. Sound familiar? The thing is, the body never truly switches off, and when your body is on high alert, your gut feels it.

So, how do you regain control? Let's take a closer look at some practical solutions.

Managing Your Workload

- **Prioritisation & Organisation:** Start each week or day by prioritising tasks. Make a to-do list that separates the "urgent" from the "important," and try to tackle things in manageable chunks. For some people this may be very easy. For others like myself, this is very difficult to do but just start! I promise it does help.

- **Delegate & Ask for Help:** Understand that you don't need to do everything yourself. Learn to delegate where possible and ask for support when you need it. Teamwork can lessen the burden.

- **Set Clear Goals & Boundaries:** Setting realistic goals for yourself and communicating boundaries clearly is essential to managing work stress. A friend of mine who works in the NHS knows this struggle all too well. She's constantly approached by colleagues asking for help, advice, and last-minute favours. Since she hadn't set specific times for when she'd be unavailable, or communicated a system for non-urgent questions, these demands would pile up, creating a steady stream of stress throughout the day. It wasn't until she set clear boundaries—letting colleagues know when she'd be accessible, and asking them to send an email for non-urgent matters—that she finally regained control over her workday.

This experience is a good reminder that boundaries aren't just useful inside the office; they're essential outside, too. If you have a firm end time to leave work, communicate it openly with your team. Boundaries may feel uncomfortable at first, but they're key to maintaining a healthier balance and reducing unnecessary stress.

Tip #26: Set Boundaries at Work—and Stick to Them

Creating and holding firm boundaries at work protects your time and mental space. Define when your workday ends and make that boundary clear, so you can recharge and keep stress from spilling over into personal time.

Creating Physical & Mental Boundaries

- **Switch Off & Unplug:**

  One of the best things you can do is learn to switch off when your workday ends. This means not checking emails, silencing work chats, and genuinely focusing on downtime. Set up an **out-of-office auto-reply** if you have to. Choose when the switch goes off—maybe it's in the car on your drive home or once you walk through the door. Remember, ruminating over work does NOT help - coming from an expert on it! This is ***your*** time now.

- **Work-Life Balance Rituals:**

  Find rituals that help separate work from personal life. Whether it's going for a walk after work, changing clothes, or engaging in a hobby, these small actions signal to your body and mind that the workday is over. For me, it was going to the gym, sometimes a walk, and then I'd play the guitar for an hour or so. This really helped! So, find something that works for you.

***

Getting the Most Out of Your Commute

Your commute is an untapped opportunity for self-care. Instead of dreading the drive or train ride, use it to your advantage. In the past, I was a victim to the classic doom scrolling. Consuming large amounts of short-form video and depressing news is certainly not going to help you. So let's make use of our "dead time" - those small pockets of unproductive moments throughout your day when you're waiting, commuting, or otherwise unable to actively engage in meaningful work or leisure. It's essentially "idle" time that can often be overlooked or wasted but could be repurposed for relaxation, reflection, or quick productivity boosts.

Here are a few ways to utilise "dead time":

- **Mindful Moments**
  Instead of seeing it as wasted time, use "dead time" as an opportunity to practise mindfulness. Observe your surroundings, do some breathing exercises, or use this time to reflect. It can help ground you and reduce stress, making your day feel more balanced. I would sometimes listen to guided meditations on the app Headspace or Calm, even youtube has some great videos.

- **Personal Development & Learning**
  You can make "dead time" productive by listening to podcasts, audiobooks, or educational videos. It's a great chance to catch up on topics you're interested in and learn something new. As an avid language learner, I often used this time

to learn a new language! I practised my online flashcards or listened to content in the language. I think the main thing is to find something you actually enjoy and want to listen to or learn.

- **Planning & Organising**
  If absolutely necessary, you can use this downtime to plan your day or week, organise your tasks, or write out a quick to-do list. This can help you feel more in control and make the rest of your day more efficient. However, for me, I wanted the commute itself to be a relaxing part of my day, so I would plan elsewhere. But this could still work for some people.

- **Relax & Unwind**
  Not all dead time needs to be productive. If your day is usually packed, these moments are perfect for a quick mental break. Listen to your favourite music, read a novel, or simply enjoy the moment without feeling the need to be "doing" anything. Occasionally, I would just sit on the train without a book, a phone or anything, like an absolute weirdo! Sometimes, this was the most relaxing part of my day!

By reframing these moments as opportunities for growth, relaxation, or preparation, "dead time" can become valuable moments that enhance your day rather than feeling like wasted time. I actually ended up looking forward to the commute because it meant I had valuable “me” time. And so, by intentionally using dead time to relax, prepare, or reflect, you shift your mindset away from idle waiting and into mindful, meaningful activity.

So, next time you find yourself in one of these moments—whether it's a commute, waiting in line, or even a pause between meetings—try to approach it with intention, and you'll find that even these small snippets of time can make a big difference to your overall stress and well-being.

Tip #27: Use 'Dead Time' as an Opportunity to Unwind

Transform downtime, like your commute or waiting times, into moments for relaxation or growth. Listen to music, practise mindfulness, or enjoy an audiobook to reduce stress before or after work.

Cultivating Self-Care & Stress Management at Work

In the chaos of deadlines and to-dos, self-care at work often takes a back seat. But weaving in a few simple habits throughout your day can make a huge difference. By adding movement, eating well, and practising mindfulness, you're not just managing stress—you're building resilience. Here are some easy strategies to integrate self-care into your workday:

- **Take Breaks & Move**: Short breaks, stretching, or a quick walk can help reset your energy.
- **Eat Well & Hydrate**: Keep healthy snacks on hand, stay hydrated, and moderate caffeine (more on that in Chapter 12, page 313).
- **Practise Mindfulness at Your Desk**: One thing that really helped me was setting three alarms throughout the day to remind myself to be present. Each alarm gave me a moment to either do a short breathing exercise or engage in a 3-minute meditation using one of my apps. It was a turning point for me, offering a quick reset and reducing stress significantly. I'm certain this simple practice could work wonders for you, too.

Small changes can add up to big relief, making your work life more balanced and sustainable.

Learning to Say "No" with Confidence

Many people struggle with saying "no," especially in a work environment. I used to find myself in the same boat, always agreeing to take on more tasks, attend extra meetings, and deliver last-minute presentations because I didn't want to let anyone down. But guess what? It led to me feeling overwhelmed and, ultimately, burned out. It wasn't until I learned how to assert myself and confidently set boundaries that I started feeling more in control of my workload and my time.

The good news is, saying no doesn't have to be confrontational or rude. It's about being clear and honest while maintaining a sense of control over your time. It's about being able to say no while still being polite and professional. When done well, saying no can actually make you feel more confident, respected, and capable.

Here's how to do it:

- **Be Direct but Polite**: Keep it simple and straightforward without over-explaining. For example: *"Thank you for thinking of me, but I won't be able to take this on right now."*
- **Offer Alternatives (if appropriate)**: If you genuinely want to help but don't have the capacity, suggest an alternative. *" I'm not available to assist with this today, but I could help out next week."*
- **Use "I" Statements**: Frame your response around your own workload and priorities to prevent any misunderstanding of your intentions. *"I'm currently focused on a deadline, so I won't be able to commit to this task."*
- **Practise Saying No to Build Confidence**: Like any skill, it takes practice. Start small with low-stakes scenarios to build up your confidence.
- **Set Boundaries with Assertiveness, Not Aggression**: It's okay to prioritise your well-being. Being assertive, not aggressive, will help you set boundaries that support both your productivity and peace of mind.

If the phrases above weren't enough, here are some additional strategies to say "No" clearly & kindly:

- **Show Gratitude Before Declining**:
  "I appreciate the offer, but I'm currently unable to commit to this."

- **Highlight Current Commitments**:
  "I'm at capacity with my current projects and won't be able to assist with this one."

- **Defer with a Positive Spin**:
  "This sounds like a great opportunity, but I'll need to pass this time."

- **Suggest Checking Back Later**:
  "I'm unavailable right now, but please check back with me in a couple of weeks."

- **Ask for More Information (When You're Unsure)**:
  "Before I commit, could you let me know the expected timeline and details? I want to make sure I can fully dedicate myself to it."

- **Empower the Requester to Make a Decision**:
  "I can help with this task, but it would mean pushing back on X project. How would you prefer I proceed?"

- **Point Out Overlap with Your Role/Expertise**:
  "I believe [colleague's name] is more suited for this task given their expertise."

Tips for Politely Declining in Different Contexts:

- **When Asked to Join a Meeting**:
  "Thank you for including me. However, my current schedule is packed, and I may not be able to contribute as much as I'd like. Could you send me the notes afterwards instead?"

- **When Asked for Your Time Last-Minute**:
  "I would love to help, but I need more notice to accommodate this in my schedule."

- **If Someone Requests an Unreasonable Deadline**:
  "Given my current workload, I won't be able to complete this by [date]. Would [alternative date] work for you?"

In my experience, once I became more comfortable with saying no, my workload significantly lightened, and I felt more in control of my time. My stress levels dropped, and I actually became more productive because I was no longer stretched too thin.

Tip #28: Practise Saying 'No' Confidently and Kindly

Use clear, polite language to set limits on your workload. Saying no when necessary allows you to protect your time and energy for tasks that align with your goals.

By setting boundaries and learning to say no confidently, you not only protect your time but also improve your self-respect and confidence. You become the one who directs your workload rather than letting it overwhelm you.

The Work-Life Balance Myth

We hear it all the time, "achieve balance, and you'll find happiness and reduce stress." But when it comes down to it, trying to maintain a perfect work-life balance can feel like juggling flaming swords while walking a tightrope—and someone's just thrown in a few chainsaws for good measure.

Life is messy, work is demanding, and sometimes it all feels like trying to keep a houseplant alive—one day, it's thriving, the next it's a wilted mess because you "forgot" to water it (again). And much like houseplants, the reality is that work and life won't ever stay perfectly balanced for long; they'll always tilt one way or the other.

Reframe the Myth of Balance

Instead of striving for some fairytale "balance" where work never spills into your life or vice versa, think about *integration*. This isn't about forcing everything into neat little boxes—rather, it's about *flow*. Some days, work takes the lead; other days, your personal life demands your focus. The key is to be flexible, adjust as needed, and stop holding yourself to an impossible standard.

"Balance is not something you find, it's something you create."

Jana Kingsford

Let's face it: striving for a picture-perfect balance can actually add more pressure when it feels unattainable. The point isn't to feel guilty every time you're working late or spending a day binge-watching Netflix. It's about recognising that, sometimes, work will demand more of you, and other times, life outside of work will take precedence—and that's okay.

Balance Doesn't Mean Equal, It Means Manageable

The true aim is to make sure you don't tip the scale so far in one direction that you're about to tumble over. It's more like learning how to surf: sometimes, you're catching the perfect wave, and sometimes, you're tumbling headfirst into the ocean. You'll find yourself paddling furiously some days, and others, you'll be calmly coasting along. *That's balance.*

Work-Life Integration: The Realistic Approach

Forget the scale and start thinking about work-life integration. How can you weave work and life together in a way that reduces stress? It might look like taking a 10-minute walk outside during your workday to clear your mind, or it might mean dedicating 30 minutes at night to something you genuinely love doing. Remember, it's not about having two separate, perfectly balanced buckets called "Work" and "Life"—it's about finding what feels right to you.

So, let go of the guilt, embrace the chaos, and focus on what brings you joy, peace, and a sense of fulfilment. And, for the love of all things sacred, stop trying to be a juggler. Let those flaming swords hit the floor once in a while—it's far more entertaining anyway.

The Art of Prioritisation: Don't Let Your To-Do List Be the Boss of You

We've all been there—the moment you look at your workload and it feels like a mountain, growing taller with every passing hour. But guess what? You don't need to scale Everest in one go; you just need to figure out where to place your foot first. That's where the art of prioritisation comes in.

One trusty tool for cutting down the chaos is the *Eisenhower Matrix*, a simple yet powerful way to categorise tasks based on two factors: urgency and importance. Imagine a grid: on one side, tasks are either urgent or not, and on the other, important or not. You'd be surprised at how much you can eliminate once you realise not everything is *both* urgent *and* important. Prioritise the important stuff, delegate the less critical, and save the "can-wait" tasks for, well... later.

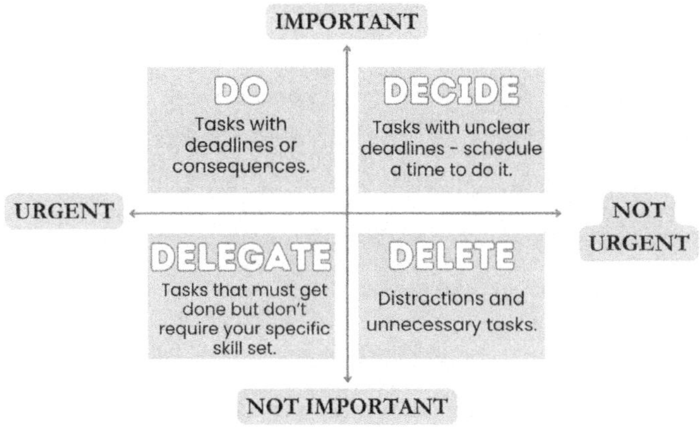
IMPORTANT
DO
Tasks with deadlines or consequences.
DECIDE
Tasks with unclear deadlines - schedule a time to do it.
URGENT
NOT URGENT
DELEGATE
Tasks that must get done but don't require your specific skill set.
DELETE
Distractions and unnecessary tasks.
NOT IMPORTANT

The Two-Minute Rule: Your Quick Win

A great rule of thumb to help conquer that avalanche of tasks is the *Two-Minute Rule*: if a task takes less than two minutes, just do it. Seriously. It's like swatting flies—if you let them buzz around for too long, they'll just drive you crazy. And those quick wins add up; knocking off tiny tasks gives you a sense of progress and clears mental space for the bigger stuff.

Break It Down Like a Pro

Got a bigger project that feels like it's going to eat you alive? Break it down. Think of it like building a Lego masterpiece—each small piece you snap into place eventually forms the whole picture. Chunking large tasks into smaller, more manageable actions makes it easier to start, helps prevent overwhelm, and gives you more opportunities to feel accomplished as you check things off. Remember, the idea is to make your workload work for *you*. Prioritise, simplify and take it one small step at a time.

Perfectionism at work

We've already explored the downsides of perfectionism in a broader context, but when it comes to work, perfectionist tendencies often come into sharper focus. At work, perfectionism can manifest as constantly tweaking presentations, over-preparing for meetings, or feeling the need to triple-check every email. While this drive for excellence may win some accolades, it can also be a source of relentless stress, making you feel like you're running a marathon on a hamster wheel.

In my own experience, this kind of perfectionism made my days longer and my stress levels higher. And guess what? It didn't make my work better—it just made me more exhausted. When you're constantly aiming for an unreachable standard, the pressure can snowball, affecting your mental well-being and, for those of us with IBS, amplifying symptoms.

Tip #29: Prioritise Progress Over Perfection

Accept that not every task requires flawless execution. Focus on completing work to a high standard without getting lost in endless adjustments, allowing you to move on and avoid burnout.

Striking the Balance: Excellence vs. Perfection

Here is the thing to remember. Excellence and perfection are not the same. You can deliver excellent work without the endless polishing that comes with a perfectionist mindset. This means learning to recognise when "good enough" is, in fact, great. Ask yourself: does this task need to be flawless, or is it more important to get it done efficiently and move on?

Celebrate small wins along the way. It's easy to overlook the progress you're making when you're caught in the cycle of perfectionism. But consistent, quality work is often far more valuable than striving to attain perfection every single time.

In the context of work stress, embracing a mindset of "progress over perfection" will not only protect your mental health but will also make you more efficient and effective in your role. Your time is valuable, and sometimes, "good enough" is just what you need to free yourself from the shackles of perfection.

Physical and Mental Boundaries: Making Your Workspace Work for You

Your workspace is more than just a place to plop your laptop and get on with it. It's a space that can either lift you up or drag you down—and it's all in how you shape it. The goal is to create a physical and mental boundary that helps you find that "sweet spot" between being productive and not feeling like your work is sneaking into every corner of your life.

The Physical Space – Choose Wisely, My Friend

Working everywhere and anywhere may sound efficient, but it can quickly turn every inch of your house into a reminder of emails, deadlines, and never-ending to-do lists. Been there, done that. Trust me, it's not fun. For ages, I worked in every room of my house—even my bedroom, especially during Covid—and it felt like I couldn't escape. Suddenly, my bed, which is meant for relaxing and sleeping, started to scream "spreadsheet" and "Zoom meeting."

It wasn't until I designated one corner of a room as my workspace that things began to change. My productivity went up, and my stress levels went down. And guess what? My bedroom became a sleep sanctuary once more. Now, when I walk away from my desk, it's like closing the door on work, mentally and physically.

So pick a corner, a desk, a chair—whatever you have—and make it your work HQ. Tidy it up, add a plant, get a decent chair, and use good lighting (natural light is your friend). This is your professional zone; the rest of your home is not.

Mental Boundaries – The Routines that Work (or Don't)

Now, let's talk about those mental walls. Just because you've got a desk doesn't mean your brain automatically knows when to work and when to chill. You need to build mental "on" and "off" switches. For me, setting alarms throughout the day was a great way. Every few hours, I'd get a gentle reminder to either be present, take a quick breathing break, or do a short meditation. It's amazing how just a 3-minute pause can reset your entire day.

Routines are your friend here. Get up, change into your work clothes (yes, real clothes—no pyjamas), and start your day with something intentional—a cup of coffee, a walk around the block, or blasting your favourite tune. At the end of the workday, do the same. Change your clothes again, go for another walk, or play that song that screams, "I'm off the clock!"

A Clear "On" and "Off" Switch – Keeping the Balance

When you have these physical and mental boundaries, your brain is more likely to cooperate. Your body knows when to work, and it knows when to rest. It's like Pavlov's dog but in a way cooler, less weird way.

Take these steps, and suddenly, work isn't the all-consuming monster it might feel like now. It has its time, and then, so do you. And when it comes to stress management, that separation—those boundaries—can make a world of difference.

So, next time you're tempted to bring your laptop into bed, remember this: your bedroom should be your sanctuary—a place for sleep, relaxation, and everything that recharges you. By setting those boundaries, you'll create a clear divide between work and rest, helping your mind and body know when to power down and when to switch on.

Tip #30: Use Recovery Time to Recharge, Not Just Rest

When you step away from work, make sure your downtime actually serves to recharge you, not just occupy time. This means opting for activities that actively relax and energise you—like going for a walk, reading a book, or practising mindfulness—rather than just zoning out with TV or social media. True recovery is what helps you return to work with a refreshed body and mind.

Mindful Moments at Work

Sometimes, work stress hits hard and fast—like an unexpected email, a last-minute deadline, or just that creeping overwhelm that builds throughout the day. When that happens, taking a "micro-break" can work wonders. These tiny pauses don't have to be complicated, but they do need to be intentional. Start with mindfulness exercises that are designed to ground you right in that moment: focus on your senses—what do you see, hear, touch, taste, and smell? Centering your awareness can quickly calm racing thoughts and help you regain focus. It's almost like hitting the mental "reset" button.

In addition, stepping away from your screen for a moment can be incredibly refreshing. Stretch your arms, roll your shoulders, walk around, or just take a few deep breaths. Even just standing up and looking out of a window can provide a moment of stillness in the chaos of a busy workday. Remind yourself: "This too shall pass."

This powerful reminder comes from a story I first read in the incredible (and highly recommended) Eckhart Tolle's *A New Earth*. It's about a king who sought a phrase that would be equally relevant in both the best and worst of times. One of his advisors presented him with a ring inscribed with the words "This too shall pass." The king found comfort in it during difficult times and humility during joyful moments, as it reminded him that every experience, whether good or bad, is fleeting. So when the workday feels overwhelming, or when stress levels skyrocket, repeating this phrase can help ground you, offering a perspective of acceptance and balance. If it wasn't for my fear of getting tattoos, I would probably get this phrase across my arm!

By acknowledging that even the most intense moments are temporary, you allow yourself to regain perspective and find calm amidst the storm of your workday. Remember, taking these small moments to pause and breathe can have a significant impact on managing stress in the moment.

Another useful grounding phrase to remember comes from Ryan Holiday's book, *The Obstacle is the Way*. One that resonates in times of stress is, **"This moment isn't your life, it's just a moment in your life."** It's a powerful reminder that whatever stress or obstacle you're currently facing is temporary. Let that thought guide your breathing—inhale, knowing this is just a moment, and exhale, letting the stress pass through and away from you.

Remember Your Tools: Grounding and Breathing

Throughout the book, we've discussed grounding exercises and breathing techniques like the 7/11 breath (inhale for 7 seconds, exhale for 11) and box breathing (inhale for 4, hold for 4, exhale for 4, hold for 4). When stress comes, these are your go-to strategies. Remember to set a 3-5 minute timer while doing it too. Grounding helps to bring you back to the present, stopping your mind from spiralling. As I'm sure you're aware by now, breathing techniques calm your nervous system, help release tension, and make you feel centred. When work gets overwhelming, remember: these tools are always with you, ready to help you navigate any moment of stress.

Handling Work Conflicts and Relationships

Let's not deny it—work isn't just about tasks, deadlines, or responsibilities. It's about people. And sometimes, those people make it challenging to get through your day without an eye roll or a sense of dread. Work conflicts, whether they come in the form of power struggles, personality clashes, or competing interests, are all part of the modern workplace. But navigating these conflicts effectively can have a significant impact on your stress levels and, of course, your IBS symptoms.

When Work Feels Like a Battlefield

Think of it like this: You're trying to sail through your workday, but sometimes it feels like you're surrounded by stormy seas, sharks, and the occasional pirate—only they're your colleagues or boss. I've been there. In one of my previous roles, I felt like I was dealing with a "King Nero of the office"—a boss whose every whim needed to be followed and whose expectations were ever-changing. This individual had an aura of control that spread fear and intimidation through the team. I was constantly on edge, second-guessing myself, and bending over backwards to avoid confrontation. The stress of dealing with that dynamic spilled over into my personal life, and my IBS symptoms flared up big time. It felt like I was living with a constant knot in my stomach.

In those moments, it became crucial to learn the art of navigating difficult work relationships.

Strategies for Navigating Work Conflicts

Conflicts are inevitable, but they don't have to be explosive. Approaching disagreements calmly and openly, without making it personal, can defuse tension before it boils over. Instead of jumping to conclusions or becoming defensive, focus on understanding the other person's perspective. When I was dealing with "King Nero," I found that asking clarifying questions—"Can you help me understand what you're looking for here?"—helped soften their approach and made it easier for both of us to communicate.

Setting Professional Boundaries

For a long time, I let people invade my work and personal space. Staff would wander into my classroom during planning time, and my desk felt more like a communal space than my own. At first, it felt impossible to say, "Actually, I need this time to plan" without feeling guilty. But I soon learned that setting respectful yet firm boundaries is key to protecting your mental energy. Assertiveness isn't about being rude; it's about valuing your time and letting others know how they can respect it.

Example Tip: Practise saying things like, *"I'm currently in the middle of planning, but let's find another time to talk."*

Dealing with Gossip, Secrets, and Hidden Agendas

It's one thing to deal with direct conflicts, but what about those murky waters of office politics—gossip, secrecy, or backhanded comments? These interactions can be just as draining. The best way to navigate this toxicity is to choose not to engage. Don't be afraid to step away from conversations that are unprofessional or damaging, and don't feel pressured to get involved in the drama.

In one job, I found myself in an environment rife with gossip and whispers. It seemed like everyone had an opinion about everyone else. And while it was tempting to listen or chime in (we're all human, right?), I found that distancing myself kept my stress levels down. I learned to focus on my work and not get drawn into the negativity.

Practise Compassion—Even When It's Tough

Easier said than done, right? But here's the thing: Everyone's struggling with their own challenges. Your overbearing colleague may be going through a rough patch, or that rude email might have been a reaction to their own stress. Practising empathy can help put things into perspective and make conflicts feel less personal. Sometimes, just understanding that everyone's fighting their own battles can make the workplace a little easier to bear.

In fact, I had an eye-opening experience in one of my jobs with a colleague I thought was out to sabotage me. After one particularly heated conflict, we ended up having a heart-to-heart, and I discovered that they were going through some really tough personal issues. It made me realise that so much of their behaviour was a reflection of their struggles—not necessarily a direct attack on me. We managed to rebuild trust, and now, believe it or not, we're still friends to this day.

Transforming Toxic Dynamics

When faced with toxic relationships, it's easy to feel trapped. But once you recognise that you have options, it becomes easier to approach these dynamics proactively. Sometimes that means having a difficult conversation to address the issue; other times, it may mean stepping back and not allowing someone's negativity to dictate your mood or self-worth.

A colleague I worked with would often vent in my space, unloading frustrations on me that had nothing to do with my role. In fact, this happened with multiple people doing this every single day. It took a long time, but I finally found the words: "I understand you're feeling stressed, but I need to focus on my work right now." The first time saying it felt awkward, but the relief afterward was like a weight lifted from my shoulders!

Detaching Your Self-Worth from Work Conflicts

It's easy to get caught up in the emotional whirlwind of work drama, but remember this: your self-worth is not tied to your work relationships. When I found myself overthinking conflicts or feeling anxious about work politics, grounding myself and remembering that I was more than my job helped me regain perspective. Focus on what you can control, let go of what you can't, and understand that people's behaviour often has more to do with them than with you.

Work conflicts are bound to happen, but they don't have to control your emotional well-being. With the right strategies and boundaries in place, you can navigate difficult dynamics and maintain your peace of mind. Remember, at the end of the day, it's not about avoiding conflict but learning to manage it effectively so that your health and happiness are protected. And that's worth more than any workplace drama ever could be.

Redefining Your Relationship with Work

One of the most transformative ways to manage work stress is by understanding why you work in the first place. What is it that drives you? What do you value about your career? As Howard Thurman[1] said, “Don’t ask what the world needs. Ask what makes you come alive, and go do it. Because what the world needs is people who have come alive.” When you align your daily work with what makes you feel alive and purposeful, your role feels less like a burden and more like a meaningful contribution to your life and those around you.

Ask yourself: “What do I want to achieve in my job beyond the paycheck?” Whether it's learning new skills, contributing to a team effort, or supporting your family, clarifying your "why" helps you navigate stress with a sense of purpose. It’s about finding deeper fulfilment in what you do, which makes all the difference in how you approach your work and your well-being.

Here are some powerful questions to help you dive even deeper into your purpose and values:

- If money and status were no object, what would I do?
- If I were less afraid of other people's opinions, what would I say?
- What actually makes me happy?
- Does success make me happy?

---

1. Howard Thurman (1899–1981), a key mentor to Martin Luther King Jr., was a prominent African American theologian, philosopher, and civil rights leader, known for his advocacy of nonviolence and spiritual transformation.

- What is my definition of success if money were taken out of the equation?
- What are the things that I'm hiding from myself?
- What are the emotions that I'm unprepared to feel?

Finding Fulfilment Beyond Work

But work is just one chapter in the book of life. When the only joy or validation you get comes from your job, work becomes a much larger source of pressure. Finding hobbies, nurturing relationships, and exploring interests outside of work can help you achieve a sense of fulfilment that doesn't hinge on your career. I once found myself obsessing over work, believing it was the be-all and end-all of my identity. But once I started cultivating friendships, rediscovering my love for music, and finding joy in simple activities like cooking or going for a walk, I realised how important it was to seek balance beyond the office.

When Work Stress Feels Overwhelming

Sometimes, despite your best efforts to manage stress, it feels like work is all-consuming. If that's the case, reaching out for support is not just a good idea—it's essential. Seeking help from a counsellor, stress management coach, or even talking to your HR team can make a world of difference. It's okay to admit that you're struggling and need guidance; this step can be pivotal in regaining control over your mental health.

And then, there may come a time when you need to recognise that your current job or environment is no longer serving you. If stress persists despite all your efforts, it may be time to consider a change—whether that means exploring new opportunities within your organisation, finding a different role that aligns better with your values, or even taking a break to focus on your health. Remember, you are not stuck. You always have choices, even if they're difficult ones.

Ultimately, work is a marathon, not a sprint. It's about adopting sustainable habits, setting healthy boundaries, and prioritising self-care—all crucial to maintaining long-term well-being. When managed with intention, work can be a place of growth, fulfilment, and connection rather than a source of endless stress. Striking a balance between the inevitable demands of work and consistent self-care can improve not only your work performance but also enhance your overall well-being and happiness. Remember, you have the power to rewrite your relationship with work, shaping it in a way that uplifts, rather than drains, you.

Reflection and Practical Step

Managing Work Stress and IBS

Work is one of life's biggest stress magnets, and if you're dealing with IBS, it can feel like it's dialling up those symptoms to max volume. By stepping back to identify what really gets to you at work and exploring practical ways to handle it, you can start to ease that constant pressure. Let's focus on setting boundaries, spotting triggers, and making small, smart adjustments that pack a punch in managing your work stress and supporting your well-being.

Exercise: Reflection on Work Boundaries and Stress Triggers

Prompt 1: Reflection on Work Boundaries
Reflect on your current boundaries at work. Do you find yourself taking work home with you, mentally or physically? How could setting clearer boundaries improve your stress levels and, in turn, your IBS symptoms? Think about ways you can create more separation between your work life and personal life.

Prompt 2: Identifying Work Triggers
What specific aspects of your job (deadlines, workload, conflicts) trigger your stress? How do these stressors manifest in your body, especially in relation to your IBS? Reflect on ways you can either minimise or change your response to these triggers.

Practical Steps: Reducing Work Stress and Supporting Your IBS

1. **Set One Work Boundary This Week**Whether it's leaving work at a certain time, not checking emails after hours, or creating a workspace at home that separates work from relaxation, pick one boundary to set and stick to it this week.

Notice how this affects your stress levels and overall health.

2. **Take a Mindful Micro-Break**Schedule short, mindful breaks throughout your workday. These could be 3-5 minutes of breathing exercises or stretching. See how these small moments of calm affect your overall stress and help manage your IBS symptoms.

3. **Practise the Two-Minute Rule**If a task will take less than two minutes, do it right away. This helps reduce the buildup of small, nagging tasks that can create unnecessary stress and overwhelm. Notice how this simple rule helps declutter your mental space.

4. **Reflect on Your "Why"**Take time to journal about why you work and what purpose it serves in your life beyond the paycheck. Reconnecting with your purpose can help reduce feelings of burnout and stress, making work feel less overwhelming and more meaningful.

By setting clearer boundaries, practising mindfulness, and reconnecting with your deeper motivations, you can create a work environment that feels less stressful and more manageable. These actions can help reduce the impact of work stress on your IBS and bring you closer to feeling in control of your health.

Chapter 11

Rest and Digest

How Sleep Heals Your Gut

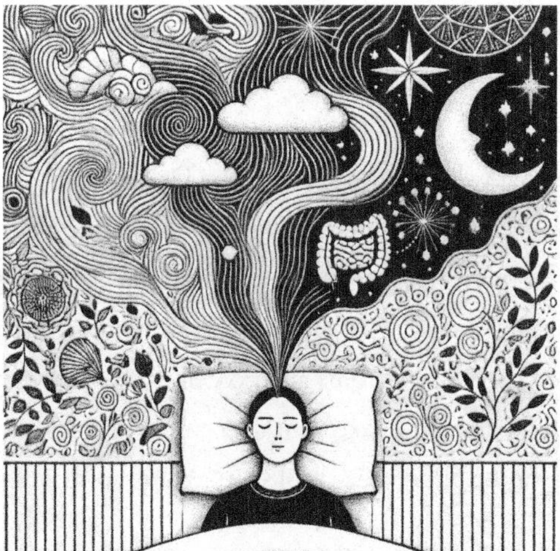

We've all experienced those rare, blissful mornings where we wake up feeling completely refreshed, like we've just conquered the world in our sleep. Unfortunately, for many of us, those mornings are few and far between. I'll be honest—I knew all the "rules" for a good night's sleep. I mean, who doesn't? But it took me years to actually stop and say, "You know what? I'm going to actively try and improve my sleep." And I did this because I was simply tired of being tired. I was sick of walking around like a zombie. I couldn't focus; my energy was all over the place. I didn't realise how much the lack of sleep was affecting my IBS symptoms (among other things!) until I finally committed to taking my sleep seriously.

***

The Hidden Impact of Poor Sleep

The truth is, sleep deprivation isn't just about feeling groggy—it's much deeper. According to sleep expert Dr. Matthew Walker, who wrote *Why We Sleep*, adults should aim for **7 to 9 hours of sleep a night** to support optimal health and function. Falling short of this can trigger your body's stress response (the "fight or flight" mode), which worsens IBS symptoms and contributes to a vicious cycle of poor sleep and increased anxiety. Walker emphasises several key points that highlight the importance of sleep for your health and well-being:

- **Sleep Deficit is Cumulative**: When you lose sleep, you don't just bounce back the next night. Walker explains that sleep debt accumulates over time, affecting your mood, focus, and overall well-being. And even if you get a solid night of sleep afterwards, it's not enough to undo the damage from lost sleep.

- **Chronic Sleep Deprivation is a Real Threat**: The body and brain don't simply adjust to getting less sleep. If you're constantly running on 6 hours when your body needs 8, you're not "getting used to it"—you're just accumulating more harm. And though you might think you're doing okay, your mental clarity, memory, and emotional stability are likely taking a hit.

- **"Catching Up on Sleep" is a Myth**: The idea that you can "make up" for lost sleep on the weekends? Forget it. A couple of nights of longer sleep can't reverse the effects of ongoing deprivation, which can include impaired concentration, memory issues, and even a weakened immune system. Plus, long-term lack of sleep increases your risk for serious health problems like heart disease and diabetes.

- **The Long-Term Consequences are Serious**: Chronic lack of sleep isn't just an annoyance; it has lasting consequences. From obesity to cardiovascular disease to a shortened life expectancy, poor sleep plays a role in numerous health issues. And again, no, getting a few extra hours on the weekend isn't going to fix it.

Tip #31: Make Sleep a Non-Negotiable Priority

So don't wait until you're totally burned out and struggling to get through your day (like I was) to start taking sleep seriously. A good night's sleep isn't just a luxury—it's essential for your mental, emotional, and physical health.

***

Practical Tips for Better Sleep

Here are some evidence-based tips:

- **Stick to a Consistent Sleep Schedule**: This is the challenging one - go to bed and wake up at the same time daily, (including weekends!) A consistent schedule helps regulate your body's internal clock, making it easier to fall asleep. I would say it's especially difficult if you have to negotiate this with your partner. Try to sit down and talk about doing a weekly trial first and then both of you will see the benefits after even just a week. This was especially difficult for me but now my wife and I have come to an agreement!

- **Limit Stimulants**: Cut off caffeine intake by early afternoon and moderate alcohol, which disrupts sleep cycles. (We will talk more about caffeine/alcohol in Chapter 12, page 356.) We know that both can impair your sleep quality and worsen IBS symptoms. For me, I was a coffee addict and had to "give up" coffee a fair few times. It reminds me of that Mark Twain quote "Giving up smoking is the easiest thing in the world. I know because I've done it thousands of times." This was especially true for me. But now that I'm caffeine-free, I sleep better, it doesn't trigger any IBS symptoms, and weirdly, my mind is clearer! It did take about a month to six weeks to work though. So, stick with it and you won't look back - I promise!

- **Create a Relaxing Routine**: Wind down with calming activities like reading, meditating, or listening to soothing music. It helps prepare your body and mind for sleep. My routine was - play calming guitar songs, then listen to an audiobook with the lights on dim. Seemed to work really well! Just make sure the book isn't too stimulating. The stories on the Calm app are especially good too!

- **Optimise Your Sleep Environment**: You've heard it all before but never do it. Here's your chance: minimise screen time before bed to avoid blue light exposure. Keep your room cool (but not cold!), dark, and quiet. I understand this can be difficult. That's why I personally invested in an "Alaska bear eye mask" I

Alaska Bear Eye Mask QR code

prefer the double strap ones (I swear by these!) and Mack's soft Ear plugs.

If you're a side sleeper I recommend the bright green ones, the "Snore Blockers". If you have small or sensitive ears the "Dreamgirl" ones or the "SlimFit" ones are your best bet". If you sleep on your back or are in a particularly noisy environment, nothing beats the original "Ultra Soft Foam Ear Plugs". I just can't use them when I sleep because I'm a side sleeper. If you're wondering, the answer is yes. I **have** tried every single type that they sell and no I'm not sponsored by them - I just used to live next to someone who seemed to enjoy listening to very loud music at 4am every night. But don't worry, she got evicted eventually!

Mack's Soft Ear Plugs QR code

- **Avoid Late Meals**: Finish eating at least 2-3 hours before bedtime to avoid sleep-disrupting digestive discomfort. If you have IBS, this is especially important to minimise flare-ups during the night. For me I would even eat 4 hours before bed to make sure it works and it definitely made a significant difference! If I had to eat later I would just eat a much smaller portion but at least give it 2 hours before bed.

Tip #32: Create a Personalised Wind-Down Routine

Establish a calming pre-sleep ritual to signal to your body that it's time to rest. Find what relaxes you—reading, soft music, or dim lighting—and make it a nightly habit. This simple routine can improve your sleep quality, reduce stress, and support your gut health.

I can promise you now that having consistently good night's of sleep will improve your resilience to stress and help regulate your digestion. Remember, it might take time to see the full benefits of better sleep habits, so be patient with the process and try to work as a team with your partner (if you have one) as it will benefit both of you. Don't be like me who had to wait 10+ years to get serious about it.

Reflection and Practical Step

Improving Sleep for Better Gut Health

Sleep isn't just downtime; it's when your body recharges, repairs, and restores itself. For those managing IBS, quality rest plays an even greater role, directly impacting the frequency and severity of symptoms. Think about your own sleep habits. Are you getting the restorative rest your gut and mind need? Or is late-night scrolling, caffeine, or stress eating into that precious time? By focusing on a few practical adjustments, you can build a routine that truly supports your body. Let's explore ways to create a sleep environment that gives your gut the rest it deserves and sets you up for a smoother day ahead.

Exercise: Reflection on Sleep Quality and Routine

Prompt 1: Sleep Quality Check-In

Reflect on the quality of your sleep over the past week. Have you been getting enough rest? How does your sleep (or lack of it) affect your IBS symptoms? Identify any patterns between poor sleep and flare-ups, and consider what changes might help you improve your rest.

Prompt 2: Evaluate Your Sleep Routine

What is your current evening routine like? Do you engage in any calming activities before bed, or are you often distracted by screens or work? Reflect on how your routine might be adjusted to create a more sleep-friendly environment. Consider incorporating relaxation techniques like deep breathing or mindfulness to help ease you into rest.

Practical Steps: Improving Sleep Quality

Choose two out of the following four practical steps to focus on. Experiment with them and see how they improve both your sleep and IBS symptoms.

1. **Set a Consistent Sleep Schedule**
   Commit to going to bed and waking up at the same time every day, including weekends. Track how this consistency impacts both your sleep quality and IBS symptoms over the week.

2. **Create a Relaxing Wind-Down Routine**
   Implement a calming pre-sleep routine for at least 30 minutes before bed. Whether it's reading, stretching, or listening to soothing music, choose an activity that signals to your body that it's time to relax and prepare for rest.

3. **Limit Stimulants and Adjust Evening Habits**
   Pay attention to your caffeine and alcohol intake. Try cutting off caffeine by early afternoon and avoid alcohol in the evenings. Also, avoid large meals right before bed, giving your body time to digest and relax before sleeping.

4. **Optimise Your Sleep Environment**
   Ensure that your bedroom is cool, dark, and quiet. Consider using earplugs, an eye mask, or blackout curtains if needed to create a sleep-friendly atmosphere that helps you fall and stay asleep more easily.

By reflecting on your current sleep habits and trying out these practical steps, you'll give your body and mind the rest they need to manage stress and reduce IBS flare-ups. Consistent, high-quality sleep can make a significant difference in your overall well-being.

Chapter 12

From Plate to Peace

Mindful Eating and Gut-Friendly Nutrition

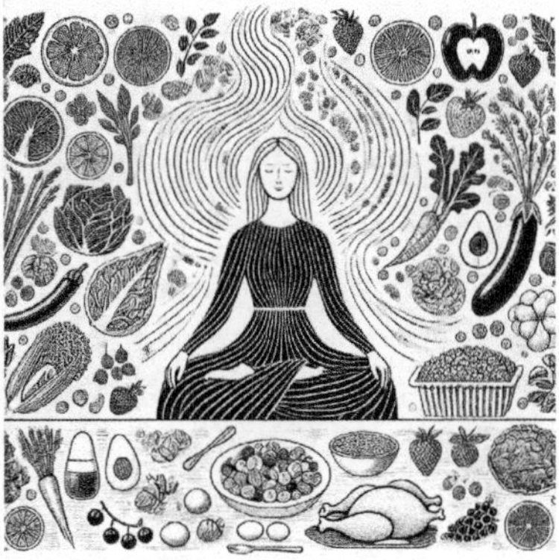

The FODMAP Diet

Food should be a pleasure in my opinion—to enjoy the wonderful tastes of different kinds of foods from around the world. When a doctor, dietician, or a book like this suddenly tells you to cut out certain foods (and drinks) from your diet, it's natural to feel resentful and to simply not do it. Welcome to the first 10 years of me living with IBS. Who are they to say I can't eat spicy food? Greasy food? Coffee? Alcohol?! Anyway, like with many other things in the book, it wasn't until a lot later (and when my condition continued to decline) that I actually started to take it seriously.

You're free to make your own adjustments, but as I mentioned in Chapter 7 (page 223), I ultimately followed the Low-FODMAP diet after trying nearly every other diet under the sun. I went through the gluten-free diet, Mediterranean,fibre-focused, even anti-inflammatory diets—all promising to be the answer for IBS. But after all the trial and error, the Low-FODMAP diet proved to be the most effective by far. It involves around six weeks of a strict elimination phase, followed by the gradual reintroduction of foods to pinpoint exactly what triggers your symptoms. While it's not a permanent solution, this process helps you understand your body's unique tolerance levels and find a diet that truly works for you. I won't sugarcoat it—it's a challenging diet and can be incredibly frustrating at times. But trust me, it's worth it 100%—and it works!

What Are FODMAPs?

FODMAP stands for a group of carbohydrates that can be troublesome for digestion:

- **F**- Fermentable
- **O**- Oligosaccharides
- **D**- Disaccharides
- **M**- Monosaccharides
- **A**- And
- **P**- Polyols

Yes, it sounds like the ingredients list for a science experiment. But don't worry—you don't need to pronounce them perfectly to know they might be causing trouble. Essentially, these are specific types of carbs that like to throw a party in your gut, but for those of us with IBS, that party can turn into a bit of a riot. While these carbohydrates are usually beneficial for gut bacteria (helping to maintain a healthy microbiome), they can ferment quickly and cause gas, bloating, and other IBS symptoms when consumed in high amounts by those of us with sensitive bowels.

So, the Low FODMAP Diet is divided into three phases: **restriction, reintroduction,** and **personalisation.** I will first focus on the **restriction phase** first, which you will need to follow for 4-6 weeks. (Experts do recommend the full 6 weeks if you can though). Yes, it will be tough, but just remember why you're doing it. Later on in the chapter, I will guide you through the **reintroduction and personalisation phases**, which are essential for increasing the variety and flexibility of your diet. It is also important to note that while FODMAPs may exacerbate symptoms, they do not harm the gut directly.

***

The Phases of the Low-FODMAP Diet

1. **Restriction Phase:** During this stage, the goal is to reduce FODMAP intake as much as possible by basing your diet on low-FODMAP foods and avoiding those high in-FODMAPs. This phase typically lasts **4-6 weeks** and allows your body time to establish a symptom-free baseline.

2. **Reintroduction Phase:** After the restriction period, you'll gradually reintroduce high-FODMAP foods one at a time to identify specific items that trigger symptoms. This phase generally spans **8-10 weeks**, as each food should be tested individually over several days to monitor for any reactions.

3. **Personalisation Phase:** Based on the findings from the reintroduction stage, you will personalise your diet to include as much variety as possible while avoiding problem-

atic foods. This is an ongoing, long-term phase aimed at supporting symptom management and creating a balanced, sustainable diet that meets your needs.

Listening to your body and adapting these phases as needed can make the process more effective and manageable.

***

Types of FODMAPs

1. **Oligosaccharides**– These include **Fructans** (like wheat, rye, onion, and garlic) and **Galacto-oligosaccharides**(found in beans and pulses).

2. **Monosaccharides**– Primarily **Fructose**, which is found in fruits, vegetables, and honey. When fructose is present in higher amounts than glucose, it is not absorbed well and may cause discomfort.

3. **Disaccharides**– This primarily refers to **Lactose**, found in dairy products like milk and yoghurt. The Low FODMAP Diet is not entirely dairy-free, as some low-lactose dairy foods can usually be tolerated in small amounts.

4. **Polyols**– These are **sugar alcohols**, like **Sorbitol** and **Man-**

nitol, found naturally in certain fruits and vegetables and used as sweeteners in sugar-free products like gum and candy.

Alright, if you're feeling ready, now is the time to jump into the 6 weeks of the **Restriction Phase** of the Low-FODMAP Diet. I know it sounds daunting, especially if you've already been through your share of diet adjustments. Trust me, I had my reservations in the beginning too.. But remember, this is a focused, temporary step to help you pinpoint exactly what's been aggravating your IBS symptoms. You'll be saying goodbye to some foods for a few weeks, but this period is essential—it's like hitting the "reset" button on your gut.

Think of this as a guided discovery phase. Yes, it can be challenging, but every meal choice you make here will bring you closer to understanding what your body needs. It's an investment in your health, and after trying other diets myself, I can honestly say it's worth it.

Okay, let's look at some foods that *are* considered low in FODMAPs:

Meat, fish and alternatives

- All meat (beef, lamb, pork, chicken, turkey, game, etc)
- Fish(fresh, tinned in brine or oil)
- Eggs
- Tofu
- Textured vegetable protein (or TVP) and Quorn mince*

- Tofu (firm and drained)
- Tempeh

Be careful of added flavours or ingredients, however, as these may contain foods on the "avoid" list. For example, *Quorn may be flavoured with onion powder. Most nuts and seeds are suitable in moderation(more information is included later regarding these).

Fats and oils

All fats and oils are low FODMAP[1] , including cooking oil, margarine, low-fat spreads, butter, ghee, lard, and suet.

NOTE: For all the details surrounding what you can and can't eat, refer to ***Appendix B****. However, when you're on the go, I highly recommend using* ***ChatGPT*** *on your phone and it will guide you on whether or not you can eat something.*

So, the following table lists high-FODMAP foods and suitable low-FODMAP[2] alternatives. Take your time with it, and feel free to

---

1. Monash University (n.d.) About FODMAP and IBS. Retrieved November 22, 2024, from https://www.monashfodmap.com/about-fodmap-and-ibs/

2. Gloucestershire Hospitals NHS Foundation Trust (2023) Low FODMAP diet sheet. Retrieved November 22, 2024, from https://www.gloshospitals.nhs.uk/media/documents/Low_FODMAP_dietsheet_for_website_Feb2023_update.pdf

keep going back to it (as it does get confusing). These recommendations have been carefully compiled from reputable sources to ensure their accuracy. Feel free to explore these sources for more detailed information or additional guidance[3].

Moderate FODMAP containing foods

Some foods higher in FODMAPs, as identified by reputable resources, can be included during the restriction phase but only in small amounts and one food at a time. For a detailed list of these 'moderate' FODMAP servings and the suitable amounts, refer to ***Appendix C***. You do not need to include these foods but can choose to if it is helpful.

From my experience, the first two weeks are the most difficult by far. Just finding out what you can and can't eat gets frustrating and annoying but I promise it does get easier and it is worth it. To help you, there are some fantastic recipes that I have used on the Monash website here: Low FODMAP Recipe (scan QR code).

You can also download their app: Monash FODMAP Diet (scan QR code).

Monash University is a leading research institution and one of the most trusted sources for testing and classifying foods as

3. For detailed guidance on the Low FODMAP diet phases, refer to Monash University's official resources.

low or high FODMAP. They pioneered the Low FODMAP Diet and continue to provide valuable research, which is why I recommend their app.

I do use the app a lot and highly recommend it if you have the means to. However, the app does cost £7.99 so an alternative (like I mentioned above) would be to just check with ChatGPT. I did this often, and it actually comes up with some really great recipes too. Give it a go!

For even more resources, I highly recommend exploring:

- FODMAP Everyday: scan QR code for tips, recipes, and expert advice.
- A Little Bit Yummy: scan QR code for dietitian-approved recipes and practical guides.

These platforms offer incredible support to help you on your low FODMAP journey!

Tip #33: Swap It, Don't Stop It

When starting the low-FODMAP diet, it's easy to feel overwhelmed and think you need to cut out a huge range of foods, but that approach can leave you feeling restricted and frustrated. The trick is to swap high-FODMAP foods with gut-friendly alternatives. Instead of cutting out all fruits, swap apples for strawberries or use chives instead of onions. This way, you're not depriving yourself of variety or nutrients—you're just making smart adjustments. Remember, the goal is to find replacements, not to stop eating foods altogether. A balanced, varied diet is still possible and will help you feel better in the long term.

***

Low FODMAP Snacks

Also, here is a short list of some great low-FODMAP snacks that I always made sure were stocked in the house for those times when I just needed a snack!

- **Rice Cakes with Peanut Butter**: Top with a small amount of natural peanut butter (ensure no added high-FODMAP ingredients) or lactose-free cream cheese for an easy, filling snack.

- **Lactose-Free Yogurt with Berries**: Pair lactose-free yoghurt with low-FODMAP fruits like strawberries, blueberries, or raspberries.
- **Homemade Energy Bars**: Make your own using oats, maple syrup, peanut butter, and seeds, ensuring to avoid high-FODMAP dried fruits or sweeteners.
- **Popcorn**: Air-popped popcorn seasoned with salt, nutritional yeast, or herbs.
- **Carrot and Cucumber Sticks with Hummus**: Opt for a low-FODMAP hummus made from canned chickpeas (using only ¼ cup serving) or other low-FODMAP alternatives like red pepper or eggplant dips.
- **Hard-Boiled Eggs**: Simple and protein-packed, great for on-the-go snacking.
- **Low-FODMAP Fruit**: Fresh options like bananas (firm- must be unripe, so we're talking green!), oranges, grapes, kiwifruit, or strawberries are safe for snacking.
- **Rice Crackers with Cheese**: Pair rice crackers with low-lactose cheese like cheddar, feta, or brie.
- **Lactose-Free Cottage Cheese and Tomatoes**: A quick,

protein-rich snack with fresh tomatoes on the side.

- **Nut Mix (Low-FODMAP Serving)**: Almonds, walnuts, or macadamia nuts in small portions (10-12 nuts per serving).
- **Coconut Chips**: Unsweetened coconut chips for a crunchy, naturally sweet snack.
- **Roasted Pumpkin or Sunflower Seeds**: Lightly salted or flavoured with low-FODMAP seasonings.
- **Baked Sweet Potato Chips**: Thinly slice sweet potatoes, drizzle with olive oil, and bake until crispy.
- **Edamame (in the Shell)**: Lightly steamed and salted; just stick to a serving of about ½ cup to keep it low-FODMAP.
- **Dark Chocolate (in Moderation)**: Small amounts of dark chocolate (up to 30g) can be a satisfying sweet treat.
- **Plain Oatmeal or Overnight Oats**: Make a batch of low-FODMAP overnight oats with lactose-free milk or almond milk and top with low-FODMAP fruits.
- **Tinned Tuna or Salmon on Rice Cakes**: A protein-packed snack that's quick to prepare and filling.
- **Vegetable Chips**: Homemade or store-bought chips made from low-FODMAP veggies like zucchini, kale, or carrots.
- **Lactose-Free Smoothie**: Blend lactose-free yoghurts or

milk with low-FODMAP fruits like strawberries, kiwi, and a handful of spinach for a quick nutrient boost.

Low-Fodmap seasonings and sauces

When I went through the low-FODMAP diet, it was so hard to find any sauce that didn't have onions and garlic in it! You can't even buy a simple pasta sauce without these ingredients. Everything seemed off-limits at first, and I struggled to make meals taste good. So, here is a list of sauces and seasonings I found helpful to keep at home—they made sticking to the diet much easier!

Seasonings and Sauces to Try:

1. **Garlic-Infused Oil**: While garlic itself is high FODMAP, garlic-infused oil is low FODMAP because the fructans (the part that triggers symptoms) don't dissolve in oil. This became one of my go-to ingredients for adding flavour without the gut distress.

2. **Asafoetida**: It smells a bit odd when raw, but cooking it in oil beforehand mellows it out and adds a delicious, garlic-like flavour to dishes. It was a lifesaver for adding depth to meals when I couldn't use garlic. I used it nearly every day.

3. **Fresh Ginger**: I used a lot of fresh ginger in my cooking—it adds a lovely warmth and spice to stir-fries, marinades, and sauces. It's not just low FODMAP but also great for digestion!

4. **Gluten-Free Soy Sauce**: Soy sauce can be tricky because some varieties contain wheat. I used the Kikkoman gluten-free soy sauce to keep things simple and FODMAP-friendly. It's perfect for adding a savoury kick to dishes.

5. **Teriyaki-Style Sauce**: I made my own version of a teriyaki sauce using gluten-free soy sauce, fresh ginger, and golden syrup (do not use honey!). It's great for marinating meats and vegetables while staying within the low-FODMAP guidelines.

6. **Shaoxing Rice Wine**: This Chinese rice wine adds a rich, savoury depth to stir-fries and marinades. Since it's usually used in small amounts, it's considered low FODMAP, so feel free to add a splash to your dishes for extra flavour.

7. **Green Pesto (Without Garlic)**: Yes, it exists! I found a garlic-free green pesto that I used frequently. It's perfect for mixing into gluten-free pasta or gnocchi.

8. **Chives and Green Onion Tops**: These became my ultimate go-to, especially when I had to cut out onions. I felt like something was always missing from my dishes until I discovered them. I ended up using them almost every day. While regular onions are high FODMAP, the green tops of spring onions or chives are a perfect alternative for adding that familiar onion flavour—without the digestive issues.

Tip #34: Choose Your Flavours Wisely

Use IBS-friendly seasonings, like garlic-infused oil or ginger, to bring flavour without triggering symptoms. This can make sticking to the diet easier and more enjoyable.

Other Low FODMAP Seasonings and Sauces to Keep on Hand:

- **Lemon Juice and Zest**: Adds a fresh, tangy flavour to many dishes.
- **Chilli-Infused Oil**: A great way to add some heat to your food without the FODMAP triggers in raw chilli.
- **Maple Syrup**: Another great sweetener for marinades or sauces like teriyaki (but can be pricey!).
- **Mustard**: Plain yellow mustard is typically low FODMAP and can add a bit of tang.
- **Herbs and Spices**: Basil, parsley, thyme, rosemary, and oregano are all low FODMAP and help make dishes flavourful without relying on garlic or onion.
- **Rice Vinegar**: A light and tangy addition to stir-fries and salad dressings.
- **Tamari**: A wheat-free soy sauce that's also low FODMAP, which you can use as an alternative to regular soy sauce.

- **Miso Paste**: I ended up using this a lot. Some varieties of miso paste are low FODMAP in small amounts and can add a savoury umami flavour to soups and dressings. I would just put a spoonful into my soup or sauce, and it made it taste great.

Okay, good luck with the restriction phase! This next stretch won't be easy, but remember why you're doing it: to finally get the answers your gut's been demanding. Keep in mind that it's just a few weeks, and every meal is a step closer to understanding what truly works for your body. There'll be ups and downs, but stay the course—you're building a foundation for long-term relief. Take it one meal, one day at a time, and remember: you've got this!

Tip #35: Commit to the Process, Not Perfection

The low-FODMAP diet is challenging. Remember, each phase is temporary and aimed at helping you understand your body's needs, so stay patient and consistent.

***

Reintroduction and Personalisation Phase

Congratulations on making it through the 6-week restriction phase! That's no small feat. Now, it's time to move forward and discover what your gut can handle. The next step—the **Reintroduction**[4] **and Personalisation Phases** of the Low FODMAP Diet—is where things get interesting.

These phases are all about identifying your personal triggers and crafting a diet that feels good and works for you in the long run. The reintroduction phase[5] typically lasts about 8-12 weeks, allowing you to systematically test each FODMAP group at a steady pace.

Reintroduction Phase

The reintroduction phase is where you'll learn which FODMAPs you can enjoy and which ones to watch out for. Testing each group

---

4. Gut Health and Nutrition (n.d.) Reintroducing FODMAPs. Retrieved from https://guthealthandnutrition.com/reintroducing-fodmaps/

5. Diet vs Disease. (n.d.). *FODMAP reintroduction challenge plan*. https://www.dietvsdisease.org/fodmap-reintroduction-challenge-plan/

systematically helps you expand your food options safely, bringing more variety to your diet without causing a flare-up.[6]

Here's a step-by-step guide to follow:

Test One FODMAP Group at a Time (usually 1-2 weeks per group)

There are five main FODMAP groups you'll be testing:

- **Fructose** (Monosaccharide) - *One Food Test Required*
- **Lactose** (Disaccharide) - *One Food Test Required*
- **Fructans** (Oligosaccharide) - ***Multiple Food Tests Required***
- **Galacto-Oligosaccharides (GOS)** (Oligosaccharide) - *One Food Test Required*
- **Polyols** (including Sorbitol and Mannitol) ***Two Food Tests Required***

By focusing on one FODMAP group at a time, you can really zero in on what works for you. Spend about 1-2 weeks on each group, moving methodically to keep everything clear. For most groups, you only need to test one type of food, which gives a good indication

---

6. For detailed guidance on the Low FODMAP diet phases, refer to Monash University's official resources.

of your tolerance to that FODMAP. However, for **Fructans (an oligosaccharide), it's important to test multiple foods.** Different types of fructans—like those found in bread, onions, and garlic—can affect you in different ways, so testing each separately helps identify any specific triggers within this group.

1. Start Slow with a Single Food for 3 Days:

- For each FODMAP group, choose one specific high-FODMAP food. For example, to test Fructose, you might start with honey. For Fructans, you could try wheat bread. *(Please see below for the chart)*

- Begin with a small amount on Day 1 (e.g., 1 teaspoon of honey for Fructose), then increase to a moderate portion on Day 2 (e.g., 2 teaspoons), and a larger portion on Day 3 (e.g., 1 tablespoon).

- Record any symptoms as you go. Testing gradually over 3 days allows you to detect symptoms at different intake levels. *(See **Appendix D** for a sample record sheet)*

2. Observe Symptoms During Each 3-Day Test Period:

- Monitor for any IBS symptoms, such as bloating, cramps, or urgency. **If symptoms appear at any point, stop testing that food**, as it likely indicates a low tolerance for that FODMAP.

- If no symptoms arise after 3 days, you can likely tolerate this FODMAP in moderate amounts.

3. Include "Washout" Days (3 Days) Between Each Test:

- After testing one food, take **3 "washout" days** by eating strictly low-FODMAP foods to allow your body to reset. This period helps you determine if symptoms were from the test food or unrelated factors.

- Only move on to the next high-FODMAP food (sometimes within the same FODMAP group) or to a new FODMAP group after having at least **3 symptom-free days.** This pause is important because your body might have a delayed response, and allowing time between tests prevents any potential carryover symptoms from affecting the results of the next FODMAP trial.

4. Repeat for Each FODMAP Group, Testing a New Food Each Time:

- Follow this pattern for each FODMAP group, selecting a different food high in that FODMAP for each test. For example, after testing Fructose with honey, you might test Lactose with a small amount of milk, or GOS with black beans. For Lactose, milk is a recommended choice, as it's a common dietary staple. On Day 3, don't feel obliged to consume all of the milk in one sitting; you can spread it out throughout the day.

By the end of the reintroduction phase, you'll have a clear idea of which FODMAP groups and food types you can enjoy in moderation and which ones to limit or avoid.

Portion Guide

Think of these portion sizes as flexible suggestions. If the portions listed feel too large or too small for your usual intake, feel free to adjust them to match what you'd normally eat. Here's a simple way to personalise the portions:

- **Day 1**: Start with about ⅓ of your usual portion.
- **Day 2**: Increase to ⅔ of your regular portion.
- **Day 3**: Try a full, normal portion.

Testing Fructans

Fructans are actually a whole family of molecules that vary in size and structure, **which means they need to be tested individually.** For this reason, you'll want to challenge each fructan-rich food separately to identify your tolerance level. Choose just one food from each subgroup—if you handle it well without symptoms, you're likely able to tolerate others in that subgroup too! To view all the details about fructan-rich foods and their subgroups, see ***Appendix E***.

FODMAP subgroups

Start by picking a FODMAP subgroup you'd like to reintroduce—let's say, lactose. Then, choose a food source for that FODMAP and a starting quantity from the guide (see the example chart below for cow's milk to test for lactose). **Remember that fortunately, you only need to test *one* food per group below!** If you handle that food without symptoms, chances are you'll tolerate other foods in that subgroup just as well. Refer to ***Appendix F*** for a complete chart of foods to test from each FODMAP subgroup.

Lactose

	Day 1	Day 2	Day 3
Cow's milk	120ml	250ml	375ml
Yoghurt, plain	125g	250g	375g

Testing Foods with Multiple FODMAPs

When it comes to reintroducing foods with *multiple FODMAPs*, it's best to save them for last. Here's why: testing each FODMAP type individually first is essential to pinpoint what your system can handle. By isolating FODMAPs—such as lactose, fructose, or fructans—you'll get a clear picture of your tolerance to each one, avoiding the confusion that can arise from testing combinations too early.

Once you understand your tolerance for each FODMAP individually, you're better equipped to handle foods that contain *multiple FODMAPs*. Some combinations might still trigger symptoms, even if each FODMAP on its own is fine. For example, you might tolerate onions (fructans) and garlic (also fructans) individually, but eating them together could overwhelm your system and cause symptoms due to the combined FODMAP load. This can also happen with different FODMAP groups; for instance, combining a fructose source with a lactose source might produce symptoms, even if each one is manageable on its own.

By waiting until the end to test foods with multiple FODMAPs, you can be confident that any symptoms arise from the interaction of these foods rather than an individual FODMAP. This phased approach isn't just about discovering which foods you can eat comfortably—it's about understanding how different FODMAPs interact in real-life meals. Armed with this knowledge, you'll have the flexibility to build a diet that truly supports your digestive health.

Other possible multiple FODMAP to test

- **Fructan + Mannitol** - Mangetout, fennel bulb, sweetcorn, cauliflower, sugar snap peas
- **Fructan + Sorbitol** - Nectarine, plum, prune, blackberries,

butternut squash

- **Fructan + Fructose** - Sultanas, asparagus, Jerusalem artichoke
- **Fructose + Sorbitol** - Apple, pear
- **Fructose + Fructan + Mannitol** - Watermelon

Personalisation Phase (Long-Term Management)

If you've made it to the personalisation phase[7], congratulations—seriously! Getting to this stage is a true testament to your dedication and resilience. Now, all your hard work is about to pay off as you personalise your diet to suit your unique tolerance levels, creating as much variety and flexibility as possible without triggering IBS symptoms. At this point, you'll have a good understanding of which FODMAP groups or specific foods you can enjoy more freely and which ones to limit, putting you firmly in control of your dietary choices and gut health.

1. **Bring Back Tolerated FODMAPs**: Using your reintro-

---

7. The Gut Health Doctor (n.d.) FODMAP reintroduction phase and personalisation. Retrieved from https://www.theguthealthdoctor.com/fodmap-reintroductuion-phase-and-personalisation

duction results as a guide, gradually reintroduce the foods and FODMAP groups you tolerate well. This allows you to enjoy moderate portions of certain high-FODMAP foods without discomfort, adding welcome variety to your meals.

2. **Build a Balanced, Flexible Diet**: Aim for a diet that's both nutritionally balanced and symptom-friendly. Prioritising variety not only boosts nutrient intake but also makes your diet more enjoyable and sustainable in the long term.

3. **Stay Open to Change**: Remember, tolerance levels can evolve due to factors like stress, gut health, and even seasonal changes in your body. Be open to experimenting occasionally with new foods or adjusting portion sizes to see if your tolerances have shifted.

4. **Know Your Safe and Trigger Foods**: Keep a list of your "safe" foods that don't cause symptoms, along with any known "triggers" that you prefer to limit. This will help you navigate eating out, meal planning, and social gatherings with confidence, making long-term management a breeze.

Tip #36: Trust Your Body's Cues

During the reintroduction and personalization phases, listen to your body's responses and adjust portions or foods as needed to avoid discomfort.

The **goal of the reintroduction and personalisation phases** is to determine your individual FODMAP tolerance so you can enjoy a varied and balanced diet that doesn't trigger IBS symptoms. If possible, It's wise to work closely with a healthcare professional or dietitian to help you navigate these phases and ensure you maintain proper nutrition.

***

Mindful Eating: A Better Way to Dine with IBS

Now that you have a clearer idea of what foods work best for you, let's turn our attention to how you eat. When managing IBS, food isn't just fuel—it can be a source of comfort, a trigger, and sometimes even a source of stress. We've all been there: enjoying a meal one moment and suddenly bracing ourselves for the internal debate that follows. But imagine if there was a way to bring more calm and enjoyment to each bite. That's where mindful eating comes in.

So, what exactly is mindful eating? No, it's not about eating kale salads while chanting mantras or chewing each bite 100 times (although if that works for you, go for it!). It's really about tuning in—fully experiencing the food you're eating without distractions, and paying attention to how it makes your body feel. It's like a meditation session for your meal.

Why Mindful Eating Helps with IBS

Most of us eat on autopilot—quickly wolfing down meals between meetings, scrolling through social media, or binge-watching TV. This kind of distracted eating can lead to overeating, poor digestion, and, unfortunately for those of us with IBS, flare-ups. When you eat mindfully, you're slowing down, which not only improves digestion but also allows you to recognise how certain foods are affecting your gut.

Mindful eating can help in a few key ways:

- **Regulating Portion Size**: Eating slowly gives your brain time to catch up with your stomach. You'll be better able to recognise when you're full, which can prevent overeating (a common IBS trigger).

- **Reducing Stress Around Food**: By focusing on the sensory experience of eating, you take your mind off the "what ifs"—like "What if this meal makes my IBS worse?"—and place your attention on the present moment.

- **Better Digestion**: Chewing your food properly and taking breaks between bites allow your digestive system to work at its best. Less gulping means less gas, bloating, and discomfort.

How to Start Eating Mindfully

1. **Slow It Down**

   When you start eating, take a deep breath and set an intention to slow down. It might sound simple, but it's powerful. Put your fork down between bites, chew slowly, and focus on the taste and texture of your food. Yes, it's okay to savour that bite of food like it's the best thing you've ever eaten—even if it's just a humble bowl of rice.

2. **Check In with Your Hunger Levels**

   Before you eat, ask yourself, "Am I truly hungry?" or "Am I eating just because I'm bored, stressed, or it's simply lunchtime?" The Japanese have a fitting term for this: *kuchisabishii*, which combines *kuchi*, meaning "mouth," and *sabishii*, meaning "lonely" or "empty." It's that feeling of wanting to eat when you're not really hungry, just to keep your mouth busy—a kind of "lonely mouth syndrome." Try to tune into your body's hunger and fullness cues and be mindful of *kuchisabishii* moments. Halfway through your meal, take a break—put your utensils down, breathe, and see if you're still as hungry as when you started. This simple check-in can help you avoid eating out of habit and truly enjoy what's on your plate.

3. **Engage Your Senses**

   Bring a little curiosity to your plate. Notice the colours, smells, and textures of your food, and take that first bite slowly—how does it taste? Is it sweet, salty, sour, or bitter?

This isn't about being a food critic; it's simply about savouring each moment. You might be surprised how much richer and more satisfying a meal can feel when you're truly present with it.

4. **Avoid Distractions**

   Turn off the TV, put away your phone, and for those of you who multitask like a pro (guilty!), resist the urge to work or check emails during meals. This time is for you and your food. If you're dining with someone else, make it a point to engage in conversation and enjoy their company rather than scrolling.

5. **Pay Attention to How Foods Make You Feel**

   After going through the Low-FODMAP diet, you might already have a good grasp of your trigger foods, but mindful eating can still offer fresh insights. Notice not only how you feel while eating but also afterwards. Does this meal make you feel energised and content, or does it leave you feeling bloated or sluggish? Even when you're familiar with your trigger foods, paying attention to these subtle cues helps you fine-tune your diet, supporting ongoing well-being beyond just what's on your plate.

The Ripple Effect of Mindful Eating

It's not just about the act of eating—mindful eating has a ripple effect on your relationship with food and your body. When you slow down and pay attention to what you're eating, you might find yourself making better food choices naturally, feeling less anxious about meal times, and noticing more pleasure in the act of eating itself. This shift can help you manage your IBS more effectively by reducing the fear and anxiety that often surround food choices.

Try it for one meal—just one. See how it feels. It might not be perfect at first, and that's okay. Remember, it's about progress, not perfection, and every small step toward mindful eating is a step toward better IBS management.

Tip #37: Practise Mindful Eating

Eating slowly and tuning into your body's signals can reduce stress around food and improve digestion. By savouring each bite and paying attention to how food makes you feel, you'll be more in tune with your body and better equipped to manage IBS symptoms effectively.

A Practical Tip to Get You Started

If you're struggling to start, try this: choose one meal each day where you practise mindful eating. Set a timer for 20 minutes and try to make the meal last that entire time. This will naturally slow you down and help you focus on the experience of eating. And who knows? You might just start looking forward to these peaceful pockets of eating time in your day.

***

Gut Instincts: The Microbiome's Role in IBS and Mental Health

Are We Controlled by Our Gut Microbiome?

We like to believe that we are in control of our thoughts, moods, and energy levels, but recent research suggests that trillions of tiny organisms residing in our gut—the microbiome—might have more say in our well-being than we realise. These microbes are not just passive passengers; they actively communicate with our brain through the gut-brain axis, influencing everything from our immune response to our mental health. Scientists are starting to see that our gut microbiome might be pulling more of the strings than we ever imagined.

For those of you managing IBS, it's essential to understand that while diversifying your diet is important for gut health, this is most effective once you've identified your personal food triggers. The FODMAP diet, which we discussed earlier, helps you pinpoint which foods cause symptoms, and once you're aware of those triggers, you can begin introducing a wider range of foods to help nurture your gut bacteria without risking flare-ups.

This vast community of bacteria, viruses, fungi, and other microorganisms doesn't just assist in digestion. It plays a critical role in producing neurotransmitters like serotonin and dopamine, chemicals that regulate our mood and behaviour. It's crazy to think, but some researchers are now saying that the diversity of our gut bacteria could directly influence how we think, feel, and even react to stress. This all means that a more diverse microbiome may give us more mental and emotional resilience, which is vital for anyone managing IBS.

Here's where the idea of balance comes in—while identifying food triggers is essential, diversifying your diet afterwards is key to nurturing a healthier gut. Eating the same limited range of foods—even if they're "safe" foods—can actually limit the variety of beneficial bacteria in your microbiome. And it's this diversity that's linked to improved gut health, better digestion, and even the kind of mental resilience that makes IBS more manageable.

So, here's the big question: how much control do we really have over our gut, and how much control does it have over us? As we go deeper, we'll uncover how this intricate ecosystem within us plays a foundational role in digestion, mental health, and ultimately, in finding ways to manage IBS.

Diversity: The Key to a Healthy Gut

When it comes to gut health, diversity really is everything. A more varied microbiome is often associated with better digestion, improved immune function, and greater resilience to stress, infections, and even disruptions like antibiotics. But why is this the case? Think of it this way: each strain of bacteria in your gut has its own "job"—whether it's breaking down certain types of fibre, producing essential nutrients, or managing inflammation. The more diverse your gut microbiome, the more equipped it is to handle a wide range of tasks, ultimately contributing to overall gut health and even mental well-being.

For those of us managing IBS, nurturing gut diversity is not just nice to have; it's essential. Studies reveal that individuals with IBS often have a less vibrant and diverse gut microbiome compared to those without the condition. This imbalance, known as dysbiosis, can act like a troublemaker in your digestive system, leading to intensified symptoms such as bloating, diarrhoea, or constipation. On the flip side, a flourishing microbiome can become your strongest ally—helping your body keep digestion on track, tame inflammation, and handle stress with greater ease, all while cutting down the severity and frequency of IBS flare-ups.

However, maintaining a diverse gut microbiome requires more than just reaching for a bottle of probiotics and calling it a day. It's about welcoming variety into your diet—from prebiotic-rich fibres that act as fuel for beneficial bacteria to probiotic-packed foods that add fresh recruits to your gut army. In the next section, we'll explore these practical strategies to help you build a gut that works with you, not against you. After all, cultivating gut diversity isn't just a health tip—it's your secret weapon for taming IBS and reclaiming control over your well-being.

How the Gut Microbiome Affects IBS

So, how does the gut microbiome actually influence IBS? Well, imagine your digestive system as a finely tuned orchestra. When everything is in balance, it plays a harmonious melody, but when even a few instruments are out of sync, the whole thing can quickly turn into chaos. The gut microbiome plays the role of conductor, keeping everything running smoothly. But when this delicate balance of bacteria is thrown off—either through stress, diet, or illness—it can lead to an overgrowth of harmful bacteria and not enough of the good ones. This imbalance, or dysbiosis, has been closely linked to IBS symptoms.

Gut bacteria can influence how quickly or slowly food moves through your digestive system (gut motility), how sensitive your intestines are, and even how inflamed the gut lining becomes. If you have too much "bad" bacteria or not enough "good" bacteria, it can lead to bloating, diarrhoea, constipation, and the dreaded IBS flare-ups that seem to happen at the worst possible times.

What's even more fascinating is that the gut microbiome doesn't just affect your digestive system—it's also linked to your stress levels and emotional well-being. Through the gut-brain axis, gut bacteria communicate with your brain, meaning that stress can cause gut issues, and gut issues can amplify stress. It's a vicious cycle, one that people with IBS know all too well. But by nurturing a healthy, diverse gut microbiome, you can help break this cycle, reduce inflammation, and get a better handle on IBS.

Psychobiotics: A New Frontier for IBS Management

Psychobiotics are a fascinating and emerging area of research that directly links the gut microbiome to mental health. These special strains of probiotics have been shown to produce neurotransmitters like serotonin and gamma-aminobutyric acid (GABA), which help regulate mood, anxiety, and stress levels. For people with IBS, where stress and anxiety often trigger or exacerbate symptoms, psychobiotics may offer promising new treatment options.

So, what does the research say? Studies have shown that certain strains of bacteria, particularly from the *Lactobacillus* and *Bifidobacterium* families, can have a positive impact on both mood and gut health.

For example, one study[8] demonstrated that *Bifidobacterium longum* reduced depression and anxiety scores in IBS patients while also alleviating their gastrointestinal symptoms.

Another strain, *Lactobacillus rhamnosus*, has been found to influence the production of GABA in the brain, a neurotransmitter that helps reduce anxiety[9].

Incorporating Psychobiotics in Your Diet

So, how can you bring psychobiotics into your routine? Well, you can start with fermented foods like yoghurt, kefir, kimchi, and sauerkraut, which are rich in beneficial bacteria, including *Lactobacillus* and *Bifidobacterium* strains. Supplements containing these strains can also help, especially if you're aiming to support both mood and IBS symptoms. Remember, not all probiotics are psychobiotics—so check for

---

8. Pinto-Sanchez, M. I., Hall, G. B., Ghajar, K., et al. (2017). Probiotic *Bifidobacterium longum* NCC3001 reduces depression scores and alters brain activity in patients with irritable bowel syndrome. *Gastroenterology, 153*(2), 448–459. https://doi.org/10.1053/j.gastro.2017.05.003

9. Bravo, J. A., Forsythe, P., Chew, M. V., et al. (2011). Ingestion of *Lactobacillus rhamnosus* (JB-1) regulates emotional behaviour and central GABA receptor expression in mice via the vagus nerve. *Proceedings of the National Academy of Sciences, 108*(38), 16050–16055. https://doi.org/10.1073/pnas.1102999108

strains that have been researched specifically for their mood-boosting benefits.

By adding psychobiotics into your diet, you're taking a two-pronged approach to IBS relief: calming both the gut and mind. Experimenting with different sources, tracking your responses, and finding what works best for your unique needs can gradually bring balance to both your digestive and mental health. But psychobiotics are just one exciting piece of the puzzle. There's a whole toolkit of strategies to help diversify and strengthen your gut microbiome, each one paving the way to fewer IBS symptoms and a more comfortable, confident you.

Strategies to Improve and Diversify Your Gut Microbiome

By now, you're probably wondering, "How do I actually help my gut microbiome thrive?" The good news is that with a few lifestyle tweaks, you can significantly improve the diversity and balance of your gut bacteria, which can, in turn, help manage your IBS symptoms. Let's look at some of the most effective strategies.

Prebiotic Foods: Feeding the Good Guys

Think of prebiotics as the fuel for your beneficial bacteria. These are fibres found in plant-based foods that your body can't digest on its own, but your gut bacteria love them. When you consume prebiotics, you're essentially providing a buffet for the good bacteria, helping them grow and crowd out the harmful ones. Foods like onions, garlic, leeks, asparagus, and bananas are rich in prebiotics, making them perfect for nurturing your gut.

The key is to start slow—especially if you have IBS. Fibre can sometimes trigger symptoms, so it's important to introduce prebiotic foods gradually and monitor how your body reacts. Over time, as your gut bacteria become stronger, you'll likely notice improved digestion and fewer IBS flare-ups. However, remember that the low-FODMAP diet in the previous section limits your prebiotics temporarily. So, I recommend trying this after going through the diet.

Probiotic Foods: Replenishing the Troops

While prebiotics feed the good bacteria, probiotics are live bacteria you introduce into your system through fermented foods or supplements. Probiotics can help restore balance in your gut, especially after events that might have disrupted your microbiome, like taking antibiotics or dealing with a particularly stressful time (like IBS flare-ups).

Foods like yoghurt, kefir, sauerkraut, and kimchi are rich in probiotics, giving your gut the boost it needs to maintain a healthy balance. When adding probiotics to your diet, pay attention to how your body responds, as not all probiotics work the same for everyone. As I mentioned, certain strains, like Bifidobacterium and Lactobacillus, have been shown to help alleviate IBS symptoms, so it's worth experimenting to find what works for you. More on that in the supplements section.

So by improving the diversity of your gut microbiome, you can positively influence your mental health. Studies show that a diverse gut microbiome is associated with lower levels of stress and anxiety. Incorporating prebiotic and probiotic foods, as well as stress-relieving practices like mindfulness and meditation, can help break the cycle. By taking care of your gut, you're also taking care of your mind.

Personalising Your Approach to the Gut Microbiome

Here's the thing—everyone's gut microbiome is unique, just like our fingerprints. What works wonders for one person might not work for another, which is why personalising your approach to gut health is so important. While some people might find that certain probiotics or prebiotics offer quick relief, others may need to experiment with different combinations of foods, supplements, and lifestyle changes to see results.

Track Your Symptoms and Experiment

One of the best ways to figure out what works for you is to keep a gut health journal. This doesn't have to be anything fancy—just a place where you jot down what you eat, how your stomach feels, and any IBS symptoms you experience throughout the day. By tracking these patterns, you'll start to notice what foods or stressors trigger symptoms and which strategies seem to help.

Remember, it's all about balance. If you feel great one day after eating yoghurt, but bloated the next day after a fibre-heavy meal, don't panic. Your gut microbiome is constantly shifting, and it might take some time to find the right balance of prebiotics, probiotics, and stress management techniques that work best for your body.

The Future of Gut Microbiome Research

While we've covered a lot about the gut microbiome and its impact on IBS, the truth is that this field of research is still in its early stages. Scientists are continually discovering new connections between our gut bacteria and overall health, and some of these findings could revolutionise the way we manage IBS in the future.

Fecal Microbiota Transplants (FMT)

One of the most weird and exciting developments is the use of faecal microbiota transplants (FMT), where healthy bacteria from a donor's stool are transplanted into a patient's gut. It sounds a bit wild (to say the least), but studies have shown promising results for people with severe gut conditions like *C. difficile* infection, and there's growing interest in using FMT to treat IBS as well. I actually remember looking this up around 2012 and wondering whether this would become an option for those with IBS in the future. And while it's not widely available for IBS treatment just yet, this could have a significant impact in the future.

The Role of Postbiotics

You've probably heard a lot about probiotics and prebiotics by now, but there's another emerging player in the gut health world: postbiotics. These are the beneficial byproducts that bacteria produce when they digest prebiotic fibres. Postbiotics, such as short-chain fatty acids (SCFAs), have powerful anti-inflammatory properties and may play a key role in gut health, particularly in reducing inflammation associated with IBS.

The Next Frontier

As research into the gut microbiome continues, we're likely to see new therapies, personalised treatments, and even "psychobiotics" designed to target the gut-brain axis specifically. Imagine being able to take a tailored supplement or undergo a personalised treatment plan based on your unique microbiome profile. The possibilities are endless, and it's an exciting time for those of us looking for better ways to manage IBS.

Key Recommendations for Nurturing Gut Bacteria

There are a few ways we can nurture our gut bacteria to improve both psychological and physical health through diet and lifestyle changes. Here are some of the key recommendations *(all recommended doing after the low-FODMAP diet)*:

1. Increase Intake of Prebiotics and Probiotics:
    - Prebiotics: Include more high-fibre foods like garlic, onions, bananas, asparagus, and whole grains. These fibres feed beneficial gut bacteria, promoting a healthy microbiome.
    - Probiotics: Add some "living" foods to your diet! Fermented foods like yoghurt, kefir, kimchi, sauerkraut, and pickles introduce beneficial bacteria directly into your gut. Just a little each day can make a big difference.
2. Eat Diverse:
   A varied diet with plenty of fruits, veggies, and legumes can work wonders for microbiome diversity. They say aiming for 30 different plant foods each week can keep your gut ecosystem balanced—though it sounds like a lot, remember that whole grains, nuts, seeds, herbs, and spices all count! Don't stress the exact number—just focus on mixing things up and trying new foods when you can.
3. Reduce Processed Foods and Sugars:
   I know we all eat them but the truth is that processed

foods and sugars can encourage the growth of "bad" bacteria, throwing your gut off balance. Reducing these can help maintain a healthier microbiome. You don't need to cut them out completely—just start by making simple swaps where you can.

4. Manage Stress:
   It might seem obvious, but stress has a huge impact on your gut. Make use of the relaxation techniques in this book, like mindfulness, meditation, and regular exercise, to give your gut some relief, too. Small stress-busting habits can go a long way in supporting a happier, healthier gut.

5. Consider Psychobiotics:
   Certain "psychobiotic" strains, like *Lactobacillus* and *Bifidobacterium*, which we discussed earlier, have been linked to improved mental health, potentially helping to ease anxiety and depression. If you're looking to support both gut and mental health, trying these specific strains could be beneficial.

Final Thoughts: Take Control of Your Gut Health

Your gut microbiome isn't just a supporting player—it's the star of your health story. From keeping digestion on track to shaping your mood via the gut-brain axis, this microscopic ecosystem is a powerhouse that can make or break your IBS management journey. By embracing strategies to boost gut diversity—like eating smarter, managing stress, and making small, consistent lifestyle tweaks—you're not just soothing symptoms; you're building a stronger foundation for your overall well-being.

Remember, this journey is a personal one. What works wonders for someone else might not be the magic solution for you—and that's perfectly okay. The key is to approach it with curiosity and patience, treating your body like the expert guide it truly is. Experiment, observe, and trust yourself to discover what brings balance and relief.

The future of gut health is brighter than ever, with exciting research and innovative therapies on the horizon. But you don't have to wait for tomorrow's breakthroughs to start feeling better today. By nurturing your microbiome and prioritising small, positive changes, you'll notice the ripple effects—not just in your gut, but in your mood, energy, and overall well-being.

***

The Coffee Struggle: A Love-Hate Relationship

For most of my life, coffee wasn't just a drink—it was my entire world. I had a collection of coffee-making equipment that would make any barista jealous: a sleek coffee machine, a moka pot, a cafetière, a fancy Hario pour-over set, a Nespresso machine for when I was in a rush, and of course, a coffee grinder. I was obsessed. I'd visit coffee shops and roasters, eagerly waiting for the latest fresh batch, often getting it straight from the roaster in the morning. Coffee wasn't just my way of waking up; it was a lifestyle, a hobby, and a passion. I loved talking about it, experimenting with different brews, and savouring every cup.

And that's exactly why it was so difficult to quit.

I mean, I tried to quit *hundreds* of times—seriously, I could quit easily, but I always went back to it! Coffee was woven into the fabric of my daily life, and giving it up felt like losing a piece of myself. But eventually, I hit a point where my health was at an all-time low. I was tired of the constant IBS symptoms, the stomach cramps, the anxiety, and the never-ending trips to the toilet. I was depressed, desperate for relief, and finally ready to make some serious changes.

I figured if I wanted big results, I had to make big changes. And that's when I took it seriously.

Don't get me wrong, I still miss coffee, and I've found some decent decaf options along the way. But even then, if you're on the low FODMAP diet or discover you're lactose intolerant, things get tricky—oat milk, which I thought would be my saviour, doesn't sit well with me either. In the end, though, no matter how much I loved coffee, it just wasn't worth the pain and discomfort. There are plenty of other drinks out there that can replace that morning ritual without ruining your gut.

The Physical Impact of Coffee on IBS

As much as I loved coffee, it was clearly wreaking havoc on my body. Every time I had a cup, it seemed like my stomach was in knots shortly after. The cramps would start, followed by an urgent dash to the toilet. And it wasn't just once—I was in and out of the bathroom all day long. Coffee was like fuel for my IBS flare-ups, making me anxious and jittery, which only made the symptoms worse.

Actually, I started using coffee as a way to control my bowel movements—or at least, I thought I could. I'd drink loads of coffee in the morning just to get things moving so I could use the toilet and feel less anxious for the rest of the day. But it wasn't sustainable. The amount of coffee I was drinking would leave me with the shakes and major anxiety. It became a crutch. So let me tell you, I wouldn't recommend using coffee as medication for your gut.

It was a vicious cycle. The caffeine hit would speed up my gut motility, basically making everything move through me way too fast. I'd be sitting there, heart racing, stomach turning, feeling like I was always one step away from disaster. It took me a long time to realise just how much coffee was triggering my symptoms and amplifying my anxiety. The more anxious I got, the worse my IBS became, and coffee was right at the centre of that storm.

Why Coffee and Caffeine Are So Bad for IBS Sufferers

There's a reason coffee can be particularly harsh for people with IBS. Caffeine is a stimulant that not only wakes you up but also stimulates your gut—and for people like us, that's not always a good thing. Coffee can increase gut motility, which means it speeds up the contractions in your digestive system. If you already have an overactive gut (like many IBS sufferers do), that's a recipe for disaster. It leads to those urgent trips to the toilet, diarrhoea, and the kind of stomach cramps that knock the wind out of you.

But it's not just about the physical reaction in your gut. Caffeine also ramps up your anxiety levels, and when you're already dealing with IBS, it can feel like pouring fuel on a fire. You get jittery, your heart races, and before you know it, your mind is in overdrive, which, of course, only worsens IBS symptoms. The gut-brain axis is particularly sensitive in IBS sufferers, and caffeine throws that delicate balance completely out of whack.

But it's not just the caffeine. For some, even the acidity of coffee—whether caffeinated or decaf—can irritate the lining of the gut, potentially triggering discomfort or IBS symptoms. While decaf is often a better option, it's still worth monitoring how your body reacts.

In short, coffee is a double-edged sword for IBS sufferers. It messes with your digestion, fuels anxiety, and sets you up for a day of discomfort. Quitting may seem impossible, but once you realise how much it's contributing to your symptoms, it's a step that's truly worth taking.

The Emotional and Mental Hurdles

Giving up coffee wasn't just about the physical symptoms—it was also an emotional battle. Coffee had become part of my identity. It wasn't just a drink I had in the morning; it was a ritual, a comforting routine, and even a social connector. Whether it was grabbing a cup with friends or needing that extra boost during a long workday, coffee was deeply ingrained in my daily routine.

So, when I realised I had to give it up, the resistance kicked in. I fought it hard. Nothing else seemed to provide that same comfort, that same feeling of a reset button at the start of the day. I kept telling myself I could handle it, that one cup wouldn't hurt. But of course, it did, and I paid the price every time. The hardest part wasn't the quitting itself—it was coming to terms with the fact that I had to say goodbye to something that had been such a big part of my daily life for so long.

Finding Alternatives and Adjusting

It took me a while to finally get serious about cutting back on coffee. After trying and failing countless times, what finally made me take the plunge was reaching a point where my health just couldn't handle it anymore. The constant bathroom trips, the stomach cramps, the anxiety—it was all too much. I realised if I wanted to feel better, I had to make some big changes, and that started with coffee.

Switching to decaf was my first step. I won't lie, it wasn't the same, but it did help me hold on to some sense of normalcy without the caffeine crash. Herbal teas became another go-to, especially ginger tea and turmeric tea which not only tasted good but was also soothing for my gut. I even tried chicory-based drinks, which gave me that rich, coffee-like flavour without the side effects but didn't really suit my tastes, if I'm honest.

One of the hardest parts was figuring out how to manage my energy levels without relying on that morning caffeine hit. It turns out that better sleep, staying hydrated, and keeping a regular eating schedule did wonders for me. Once I started getting more consistent sleep and drinking water throughout the day, I noticed I didn't feel as drained. I also cut back on sugar massively. It's not a magic fix, but it's definitely better than running on coffee fumes and paying for it later.

Reflection: Was It Worth It?

Looking back, was giving up coffee worth it? Absolutely. The changes didn't happen overnight, but after a few weeks of cutting back, I started noticing fewer IBS flare-ups. The anxiety that coffee used to crank up slowly began to fade, and my gut felt calmer overall. I wasn't constantly rushing to the bathroom or feeling like I was on edge all the time.

Eliminating coffee made a real difference. My energy levels became more stable, and I wasn't stuck in that vicious cycle of caffeine highs and anxiety crashes. The long-term benefits—fewer flare-ups, reduced anxiety, and improved gut health—far outweigh the initial struggle of giving it up.

I know it's not easy, especially if coffee is a big part of your life like it was for me. But if you're dealing with IBS, cutting back or eliminating it can make a world of difference. The key is to find what works for you, whether it's decaf coffee or tea or another ritual that can replace that morning cup without triggering your symptoms. For me, giving up coffee wasn't just a decision—it was a turning point in taking control of my IBS.

***

Cheers to Change: Rethinking Alcohol with IBS

Giving up coffee was hard enough, but the thought of giving up alcohol hit me even harder. Meeting friends at the pub, beer in hand, wasn't just a habit—it was part of my identity. How could I possibly go to a pub and not drink? It felt unthinkable, almost impossible. But after a long internal battle, I finally let it go—though it wasn't without its challenges.

You see, in the past, I was a huge beer drinker with a particular love for real ales. I relished the variety, the flavour, and the camaraderie of sharing a pint with friends. But over time, I began to notice something unsettling: even a small amount of alcohol would wreak havoc on my IBS. Just one or two beers could set my stomach off, leaving me bloated, cramping, and in chaos. And the aftermath was even worse—my symptoms would flare up the next day, making me regret every sip.

Let's be honest—alcohol is merciless on the gut. For those of us with IBS, it's like throwing gasoline on an already raging fire. Alcohol irritates the gut lining, speeding up digestion in some cases and slowing it down in others, disrupting the delicate balance of your digestive system. It dehydrates your body, stripping your gut of the hydration it needs to function smoothly, which can intensify cramping and bloating. But it's not just about the immediate discomfort—alcohol's effects on the gut can build up over time, making IBS even harder to manage.

Consider this: if you're drinking 7-10 pints of beer or 1–2 bottles of wine a week, you're consuming a level of alcohol that can have serious short- and long-term consequences for your gut health. In the short term, alcohol inflames the gut lining, leading to increased sensitivity and irritation—symptoms IBS sufferers are already all too familiar with. It also disrupts the gut microbiome, reducing the diversity of beneficial bacteria while promoting the growth of harmful ones, which can trigger flare-ups.

In the long term, regular alcohol consumption contributes to a condition called leaky gut, where the lining of the gut becomes more permeable, allowing toxins and bacteria to escape into the bloodstream. This can lead to chronic inflammation, which not only worsens IBS but can pave the way for other health issues, such as autoimmune conditions.

The ongoing dehydration caused by drinking further compromises your gut, leaving you more prone to constipation or diarrhoea, depending on how your body reacts.

For someone with IBS, these effects are magnified. Your gut is already sensitive, and adding alcohol to the mix compounds the problem. Even when drinking within what's considered "moderate" limits, the cumulative strain on your digestive system can make managing symptoms feel like an uphill battle.

Eventually, I had to confront the truth: as much as I'd loved a good pint, the price my body paid just wasn't worth it anymore. Letting go of alcohol didn't just help my IBS—it gave me a newfound sense of control over my health. And here's the thing: you don't have to give it up entirely (unless you want to), but cutting back or making mindful choices can make a world of difference for your gut.

The Physical and Mental Impact of Alcohol on IBS

No matter how much I tried to justify it, the effects of alcohol on my IBS were impossible to ignore. For those of us managing IBS, alcohol isn't just a casual indulgence—it's a full-blown trigger. Let's break down why:

- **Gut Irritation:** Alcohol doesn't just irritate the gut—it bulldozes through your digestive lining, sparking inflammation and hypersensitivity. The result? A raw, unsettled stomach, sharp cramps, and discomfort that lingers far longer than the drink was enjoyable.

- **Revved-Up Digestion:** Alcohol throws your digestive system into overdrive, forcing everything to move faster than it should. This often means bloating, diarrhoea, and that dreaded urgent dash to the bathroom.

- **Dehydration:** As a diuretic, alcohol strips your body of hydration, leaving your gut struggling to function. For some, this means constipation; for others, it amplifies cramping and bloating. Either way, it's a recipe for discomfort and sluggishness.

- **Disrupted Gut Bacteria:** Alcohol wreaks havoc on the delicate balance of gut bacteria. It wipes out beneficial microbes, opening the door to more frequent IBS flare-ups and leaving your digestion in constant turmoil.

- **Mental Health Impact:** The gut-brain connection means alcohol doesn't just stay in your stomach—it hits your mind, too. What starts as a moment of relaxation often ends in heightened anxiety, irritability, or low spirits as the effects wear off. Instead of unwinding, you're left feeling more drained and uneasy.

- **Fatigue and Brain Fog:** Alcohol disrupts sleep, depletes hydration, and leaves you waking up tired and foggy. Combine this with the stress of IBS, and you've got a cocktail of exhaustion and mental strain.

These effects add up to more than just digestive discomfort—they create a ripple effect that impacts your mood, energy, and mental clarity. For me, giving it up wasn't just a nice idea; it was the only way to break free from the cycle of gut turmoil and emotional regret that followed every drink. Choosing to step away from alcohol gave me back control over my IBS and my life—and it can do the same for you. But the impact of alcohol isn't just physical—it seeps into your emotions, social life, and coping mechanisms, often making it harder to let go.

The Emotional and Social Challenges

Coming from someone who drank far too much daily and used alcohol as a crutch to suppress negative emotions, anxiety, and depression, I get it—I really do. The thought of giving it up can feel impossible, even frightening when it's become your escape, your comfort, or your way of coping. But let me tell you this: there's a better version of you waiting at the end of the journey. If you truly want to heal and feel like yourself again, this is the way to do it. I've been in the heartbreaking position of watching people drink themselves to death, and I don't want that for you—or anyone. One thing that helped me find my way out was *The Easy Way to Control Alcohol* by Allen Carr (scan QR code), a practical and transformative guide that changed how I thought about alcohol. It showed me that quitting isn't about losing something—it's about reclaiming your freedom. And trust me, the clarity and peace you'll feel on the other side is worth every step.

Giving up alcohol wasn't just a physical adjustment—it was also a social and emotional one. Drinking is often woven into gatherings, celebrations, and casual get-togethers, so saying "no thanks" wasn't always easy. Whether it was a friend's birthday or a simple night out, alcohol had become a default part of social interactions. Each time I turned down a drink, it felt like I was stepping back from the group, and I worried about standing out or explaining myself.

Link to Allen Carr's Book

There was also an emotional connection to alcohol that went beyond just social pressure. A drink after a long day had become a ritual, a way to relax and switch off. Giving it up meant finding new ways to unwind and redefining what social moments looked like. It wasn't easy, but over time, I began to appreciate the clarity and consistency in how I felt without it.

The Quiet Normalisation of Alcohol

I wouldn't say I was an alcoholic, but I did use alcohol as a crutch. When I felt anxious or depressed, reaching for a drink felt like the easiest way to zone out and escape from the emotions I didn't want to deal with. But here's the thing: I could never just have one beer. My body almost begged for more. It felt like I didn't have an off switch—there was no limit.

Looking back, I realise how easy it is to fall into that trap. So many people I know would say, "I'm not an alcoholic," and I would have said the same thing. But dependency doesn't always look like the extreme stereotypes we imagine. Sometimes, it's just using alcohol as a default way to numb yourself or manage emotions when other, healthier options feel out of reach.

Functional alcohol dependency is more common than many of us realise. People drink to cope, to socialise, to relax—but often in ways that mask deeper issues. You don't have to hit rock bottom or drink from morning till night to recognize that alcohol might be playing too big a role in your life. For me, it wasn't just about the physical toll on my IBS—it was about taking an honest look at why I was drinking and what it was really doing for me (or to me).

This isn't about labelling yourself or fitting a definition. It's about understanding your relationship with alcohol and deciding whether it's truly serving you. For me, it wasn't. Once I faced that truth, I could finally start making real changes—and it made all the difference.

Alternatives and Adjustments

When I started to at least cut back on alcohol, I experimented with alternatives that would let me enjoy the moment without compromising my gut health. If you're not ready to give up alcohol entirely, here are some tips to help reduce the impact on your IBS:

- **Choose Lower-FODMAP Alcohols:** Clear spirits like vodka, gin, tequila, and even whiskey are generally lower in FODMAPs, especially when mixed with soda water and a squeeze of fresh lime or lemon. These options are usually gentler on the gut than beer or wine, which can contain more fermentable carbohydrates and irritants.

- **Avoid Beer and Wine:** Beer, especially, is high in FODMAPs due to its barley and carbonation, both of which can lead to bloating and discomfort. Wine, while lower in FODMAPs than beer, is still acidic and can irritate a sensitive gut, especially for those prone to reflux or heartburn.

- **Be Cautious with Non-Alcoholic Beers:** While non-alcoholic beers may seem like a safer alternative, they can still contain ingredients that trigger IBS. Carbonation, barley, and FODMAP ingredients are often present, so approach non-alcoholic beers with caution if you know you're sensitive to these factors.

- **Try Mocktails:** When I didn't want any alcohol at all, mocktails were an easy choice, especially when others were ordering cocktails—it felt like a natural swap. Otherwise, soda water with lime is always a good go-to (and cheap!). Sparkling water with a twist of lemon or fresh herbs also made a refreshing, gut-friendly alternative that kept things social.

Tip #38: A Simple Step to Take Back Control Over Coffee and Alcohol

Coffee and alcohol might feel like daily comforts, but for those of us with IBS, they often come at a steep cost to our gut health. Coffee, with its caffeine and acidity, can overstimulate the gut, leading to cramps, anxiety, and urgent trips to the bathroom. Alcohol can irritate the gut lining, dehydrate, and disrupt digestion, leaving you feeling worse the next day.

If these drinks are triggers, consider the freedom that comes with new choices: try easing into decaf coffee or herbal teas to keep the ritual without the toll, and for social occasions, give mocktails a go or low-FODMAP drink options. By adjusting these habits, you're taking a powerful step toward symptom relief and reclaiming the pleasure of feeling truly well. Your gut will thank you! Don't put it off. You will be surprised with how much it can actually help you.

Reflection

Looking back, reducing and then quitting alcohol entirely has been one of the best decisions for my IBS and my mental health. The constant gut flare-ups and discomfort are no longer an inevitable part of my mornings after a night out. I'm more in control of my symptoms, and my gut feels more stable overall. My energy levels are more consistent, I sleep better, and I wake up with a clearer head—no longer battling the gut disruptions and dehydration that alcohol used to bring.

For anyone with IBS, cutting back or giving up alcohol may feel challenging at first, but the benefits to your gut health are worth it. For me, it was a step that led to greater comfort, fewer flare-ups, and a healthier relationship with my social life. I'm not here to tell you to quit drinking—I'm not going to stop you. But if you think alcohol might be affecting your stomach, gut, sleep, energy, or even your mental health, it's worth a serious think. Maybe try quitting for a week? A month? See how you feel, notice any changes, and go from there. Think about your own relationship with alcohol: is it helping you, or holding you back? What could you gain by making a change?

Reflection and Practical Step

Committing to the Low-FODMAP Diet

Making dietary changes—especially something as specific as the low-FODMAP diet—can feel daunting at first. But by taking a moment to reflect on your motivations and relationship with food, you can approach this plan with a clearer purpose. Committing to the low-FODMAP diet, despite its challenges, can be a liberating step toward managing your IBS symptoms and uncovering your unique food triggers.

Exercise: Reflection on Your Diet and Motivation

Prompt 1: Reflect on Your Relationship with Food
How do you currently feel about food? Do you see it as a source of enjoyment or as a potential trigger for IBS symptoms? Reflect on how your relationship with food has evolved since your IBS diagnosis and how this affects your willingness to try dietary changes like the low-FODMAP diet.

Prompt 2: Motivation for Dietary Change
What would motivate you to commit to the low-FODMAP diet? Reflect on the personal benefits you hope to achieve by making dietary changes. How can focusing on those potential positive outcomes help you stick to the plan even when it feels challenging?

Practical Step: Committing to the Low-FODMAP Diet

This week, take a bold step and fully commit to starting the low-FODMAP diet. Yes, it might feel overwhelming, but remember: every great change starts with a first step. Embrace the plan from the beginning, knowing that consistency will lead to real insights and help you identify your true food triggers. Keep your eyes on the long-term rewards—like gaining control over your symptoms and understanding how your body responds. Take it one day at a time, be kind to yourself, and remember that every small effort builds toward lasting relief. Sticking closely to the plan at the start will set you up for success on this journey to improved well-being.

Practical Step: Take Control, One Small Change at a Time

This week, take a meaningful step to reduce or eliminate alcohol and coffee from your routine. Start small if you need to—for example, swap one alcoholic drink for a mocktail or replace your morning coffee with a decaf or herbal tea. Focus on making mindful decisions and observe how your body responds.

If you're ready, set a clear goal: commit to a week or a month without these triggers. Use this time to explore alternatives, track your symptoms, and see how cutting back improves your gut health, mood, and energy. Remember, this isn't about deprivation—it's about discovering how great you can feel when your body and mind are working in harmony.

Chapter 13

Medications, Supplements, and the Role of Exercise

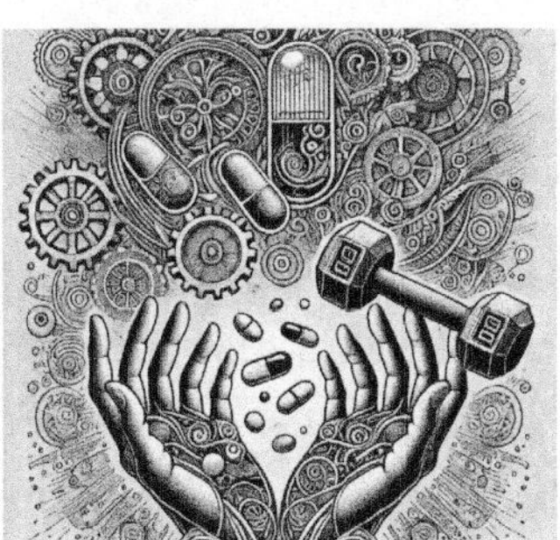

Each country has its own approach to medication, and navigating this can be tricky. If you visit your doctor with symptoms that don't have a clear cause, it's worth being cautious about taking medication right away. Of course, if it's necessary, following your healthcare professional's advice is important. In the past, I've been prescribed mountains of meds without fully understanding their impact. It's only recently that more holistic approaches have started to be prescribed—'walks in nature,' for example. Canada now has "Parks Prescriptions," and countries like Australia and New Zealand offer "Green Prescriptions," encouraging people to spend time in green spaces, gardening, walking, and generally connecting with nature.

When I was diagnosed with IBS in South Korea, I blindly accepted the pills, hoping they'd be a magic bullet for my symptoms and that I'd soon be able to live pill-free. That's the idea, right? But as you might guess, it didn't exactly go that way. The medication offered some mild relief, but it didn't fully address my IBS symptoms, and it brought along its own side effects.

It's incredibly easy to slip into a routine of taking medications like Mebeverine, Buscopan, Imodium, or laxatives, and before you know it, you're relying on them. Trust me, I've been there. Not long ago, I couldn't leave the house without my medication—especially Imodium, my anti-diarrhoea sidekick. I became completely dependent on it, finding comfort in just knowing it was there. But eventually, I started to feel like a slave to these pills, needing them to function. So, if you find yourself in a similar situation—where you can't imagine leaving the house without your meds—consider consulting your doctor about gradually weaning yourself off them and practising stepping out without them.

As I mentioned earlier in the book, for me, around 70% of my IBS was rooted in my internal world—my mindset, my focus, and my acceptance of habitual negative thinking. The rest came down to a mix of diet, external pressures, and an unhelpful lifestyle, all of which contributed to the symptoms. Keep in mind that these vague "percentages" can shift—an extended period of a poor diet, for example, will definitely tip the balance.

Managing IBS involves navigating a delicate balance between internal and external factors, which is why a multi-faceted approach is often the key to success. While mindset shifts and lifestyle changes are crucial, medications can also provide significant relief when used wisely. However, relying too heavily on medication—especially when symptoms aren't active—can turn them into a psychological crutch, limiting long-term progress. The real power lies in knowing how to integrate medications with lifestyle tweaks, stress management techniques, and dietary adjustments to create a well-rounded plan.

***

Medications for IBS: When and How to Use Them

Effectively managing IBS is a bit like juggling—you need a mix of strategies to keep things in balance. Lifestyle adjustments, dietary changes, and, when necessary, medications all have their roles to play. Medications can offer much-needed relief during intense flare-ups, but relying on them too heavily, especially when you're symptom-free, can quickly lead to dependence. The key is finding that balance—knowing when to lean on medication and when to let lifestyle and dietary changes do the heavy lifting. Here's a closer look at some commonly prescribed IBS medications and how they fit into your toolkit for a healthier gut:

1. **Antispasmodics**

   Antispasmodics, like Mebeverine and Buscopan, are commonly prescribed to relieve cramping and intestinal spasms by relaxing gut muscles—especially helpful during IBS flare-ups. I would say that Mebeverine is generally favoured for long-term, consistent cramp relief, while Buscopan is ideal for fast, short-term relief. **However, always consult with a healthcare provider to determine the most suitable option for your needs.** Here is a quick breakdown:

   <u>Mebeverine</u>

   Pros: Specifically targets gut muscles, providing cramp relief without affecting gut motility; lower risk of side effects.

   Cons: Takes time to work, so it is better suited for regular,

ongoing use.
Best for: Daily management of IBS with consistent cramping.

<u>Buscopan</u>
Pros: Acts quickly, ideal for sudden, intense cramps.
Cons: Broader action can lead to side effects like dry mouth or drowsiness; best used short-term.
Best for: Immediate relief during flare-ups.

2. **Antidepressants**
   Believe it or not, low-dose antidepressants—especially tricyclics like amitriptyline—have shown impressive results in managing IBS symptoms, particularly for those dealing with chronic pain or an ultra-sensitive gut. These medications work by tapping into the gut-brain connection, helping to balance serotonin levels in the gut and altering how the brain interprets pain signals. These changes lead to less pain, a calmer gut, and greater ease in managing IBS symptoms.

   Research Insight: Studies[1] have shown that low-dose tricyclic antidepressants can significantly improve IBS symptoms, especially when first-line treatments like dietary

---

1. National Institute for Health and Care Research. (2024, March 26). *Irritable bowel syndrome: Low-dose antidepressant improves symptoms*. NIHR Evidence. https://doi.org/10.3310/nihrevidence_62555

changes aren't enough. After six months of treatment, participants reported a notable reduction in IBS severity. This shows how these medications calm the gut's sensitivity to pain and stress. They are particularly effective for patients who have both IBS and chronic pain. But as with any medication, thoughtful use is key—**always consult with your doctor about the best approach for long-term benefits.**

3. **Antidiarrheal Medication**
   For those with IBS-D (diarrhoea-predominant IBS), anti-diarrheal medications like Loperamide (imodium) can offer quick relief by slowing down gut motility. But from my own experience, relying on these as a "fix" in every situation can backfire. For a while, I used them as a crutch—taking them before outings, even when I had no symptoms. Over time, they stopped working as well, and I'd have to up the dose just to feel secure. I also started noticing side effects from taking too many, like occasional dizziness, constant dry throat, and then the day after taking them, I would have a cycle of constipation for a couple of days after. It became a nightmare and far from sustainable.

So, while medications like these can be a lifesaver during

---

1. National Institute for Health and Care Research. (2024, March 26). *Irritable bowel syndrome: Low-dose antidepressant improves symptoms*. NIHR Evidence. https://doi.org/10.3310/nihrevidence_62555

intense flare-ups, it's essential to approach them with balance. Instead of viewing meds as the ultimate answer, take a step back and consider the broader picture—the internal and external aspects of your life that may need attention. These meds can be helpful but don't do what I did and become dependent. Take responsibility for addressing the roots of your IBS so you don't end up relying on a pill every time you go out.

4. **Other Medications**
   In addition to the options above, other medications can address specific IBS symptoms. Laxatives are often prescribed for those with IBS-C (constipation-predominant IBS) to promote bowel movements, while bile acid sequestrants are used for IBS triggered by bile acid malabsorption, helping to manage diarrhoea. Silicol gel is another option worth considering, especially for soothing flare-ups. It works by forming a protective barrier in the gut, absorbing irritants, toxins, and excess acids to ease symptoms like bloating, gas, and diarrhoea. This makes it a gentle, non-invasive addition to a broader IBS management plan, particularly for those seeking natural relief. Each of these medications targets specific symptoms and works best as part of a comprehensive treatment plan. **Talking to a doctor can help you determine the most suitable options and dosages.**

Tip #39: Use Medications as Short-Term Tools, Not Long-Term Crutches

Medications like antispasmodics and antidiarrheal pills can bring quick relief, especially during intense IBS flare-ups, but relying on them for every symptom can lead to dependency and reduced effectiveness over time. Aim to use medications as temporary aids while you work on underlying issues like diet, stress, and lifestyle adjustments.

***

Breaking the Cycle: Moving Away from Medication Dependence

As I mentioned earlier, I relied heavily on my medications for far too long—especially antispasmodics like Mebeverine and antidiarrheal pills like Loperamide. In fact, I couldn't go out without them. Even when I wasn't experiencing active IBS symptoms, I would take them preemptively, almost as a "safety behaviour." It gave me peace of mind, but looking back, I was using them as a quick fix instead of addressing the underlying issues that triggered my IBS, like stress, anxiety, and negative thought patterns.

I was viewing medication as my go-to solution rather than investing the time and effort to get better through healthier long-term strategies like relaxation techniques, positive self-talk, and visualisation.

It took time, but eventually, I made the transition. I began focusing on reducing stress and anxiety through the methods in this book rather than reaching for my meds every time I stepped out. I personally think it's important to recognise when medications are truly needed and when they're simply a comfort blanket for our anxieties.

If meds like Mebeverine and Imodium help with your stomach pain and cramps, I completely get it. I've had moments of lying on a public bathroom floor in agonising pain, thinking that anything—even a tiny bit of relief—would be a lifesaver. But it's crucial not to stop there. Tackling IBS involves a holistic approach. So now, let's explore some natural supplements and foods that can help manage your symptoms without the baggage of side effects.

Foods That Can Help IBS Symptoms Naturally

When it comes to easing IBS symptoms, whether you have IBS-C (constipation), IBS-D (Diarrhoea) or IBS-M (Mixed), another really effective approach is focusing on specific foods known for their gut-soothing properties. I have provided a list below; some things will work, and some things won't. Things that helped me a lot were taking turmeric and black pepper capsules along with turmeric tea. I also ate a good amount of fresh ginger and ginger tea. I also tried both probiotics that are on the list, I think they did help me but weren't as significant as other factors in my life – for example the low-FODMAP diet alone was like night and day for me.

Nevertheless, here is the list:

1. **Peppermint Oil**

    - *How it helps*: Peppermint has antispasmodic properties that relax the intestinal muscles, reducing cramping and easing pain.

    - *How to use*: Incorporate peppermint tea into your diet or use peppermint leaves in cooking.

2. **Ginger**

    - *How it helps*: Ginger relaxes the intestines and may ease nausea, bloating, and discomfort.

    - *How to use*: You can add fresh ginger to your meals, sip ginger tea, or incorporate ginger powder into cooking.

3. **Fennel**

    - *How it helps*: It reduces bloating, gas, and abdominal pain by relaxing the muscles of the gastrointestinal tract.

    - *How to use*: Fennel seeds can be added to dishes or steeped in hot water to make a soothing tea.

4. **Aloe Vera**

- *How it helps*: Aloe vera's anti-inflammatory properties soothe the digestive tract, potentially easing IBS symptoms like bloating and cramping.
- *Best for*: Mainly for IBS-C, to ease constipation and inflammation.
- *How to use*: Drink a tablespoon of decolorised aloe vera juice daily to avoid potential irritants.

***

Supplements to Support IBS Management

These supplements may support your digestive health and relieve IBS symptoms naturally:

Probiotics
How they help: Probiotics improve the balance of gut bacteria, which can help reduce bloating and gas and regulate bowel movements. *Best strains*:

- *Bifidobacterium infantis* (like Align): Shown to help with overall IBS symptoms, including bloating and pain.
- *Lactobacillus plantarum*: Particularly helps with bloating

and gas, especially for those with IBS-C.

Dosage: Probiotic doses can vary, but aim for at least 1 billion CFUs (colony-forming units) per serving. Here are two of the best-reviewed probiotics at the moment: Nutravita and Bio-Kult.

When adding probiotics like Nutravita and Bio-Kult to your routine, remember that results take time—you won't see an overnight transformation. It usually takes a few weeks (around 4–8) of consistent use to really feel the benefits. But stick with it, and you may notice improvements like reduced bloating, less abdominal discomfort, and more regular bowel movements. The key is patience and consistency; those small changes over time show that your gut is starting to heal and balance itself.

1. **Psyllium Husk (Soluble Fibre)**
    - *How it helps*: Regulates bowel movements by adding bulk to stool for IBS-D and softening stool for IBS-C.
    - *Best for*: Both IBS-C and IBS-D.
    - *Dosage*: Start with ½ to 1 teaspoon in water daily, gradually increasing as needed. Remember to drink plenty of water.
2. **Turmeric (Curcumin)**
    - *How it helps*: It has anti-inflammatory and soothing effects on the digestive tract, which may alleviate pain and

bloating.

- *Dosage*: 500–1,000 mg daily. Look for supplements that include black pepper extract (piperine) to enhance absorption.

3. **Magnesium**

   - *How it helps*: Acts as a natural laxative by relaxing intestinal muscles and drawing water into the bowels.
   - *Best for*: Alleviating constipation in IBS-C.
   - *Dosage*: 200–400 mg of magnesium citrate or magnesium oxide as needed.

4. **Slippery Elm**

   - *How it helps*: Coats the digestive tract with a soothing film, reducing irritation and promoting healthy mucous production in the gut.
   - *Best for*: Both IBS-D and IBS-C.
   - *Dosage*: 400 mg in capsule form or 1–2 teaspoons of powder mixed in water daily.

5. **Digestive Enzymes**

   - *How they help*: Aid in breaking down food, which may

reduce bloating, gas, and discomfort.

- *Best for*: People who experience IBS symptoms triggered by specific foods.
- *Dosage*: Take before meals; look for enzymes like lipase, protease, and amylase.

6. **L-Glutamine**
    - *How it helps:* Supports gut lining health, reduces inflammation, and may help repair intestinal damage.
    - *Best for:* Reducing diarrhoea in IBS-D.
    - *Dosage:* 5 grams daily, taken on an empty stomach.
7. **Peppermint Oil (as a Supplement)**
    - *How it helps:* Similar to consuming it as a food, enteric-coated capsules of peppermint oil relax the intestinal muscles, helping with cramping.
    - *Dosage:* 180 to 200 mg 2-3 times a day, preferably in enteric-coated capsules to prevent heartburn.
8. **Thiamine (Vitamin B1)**
    - *How it helps:* Supports energy production and nerve function, potentially benefiting the gut-brain connection and easing IBS-related fatigue.
    - *Best for:* IBS-related fatigue or low energy.

- *Dosage:* 50-100 mg daily, consult a healthcare provider for advice.

9. **Calcium Polycarbophil**
   - *How it helps:* A bulking fibre that normalises stool consistency, helping with both IBS-C and IBS-D.
   - *Dosage:* Typically 1,000 mg daily, consult a healthcare provider.

10. **Prebiotics**
    - *How they help:* Prebiotics support the growth of beneficial gut bacteria like Bifidobacteria, which can be particularly helpful for those with IBS. However, some prebiotics, such as inulin, can cause discomfort or diarrhoea (I experienced this myself), so starting with gentler options like galacto-oligosaccharides (GOS), partially hydrolysed guar gum (PHGG), or pectin is often better tolerated.
    - *Best for:* Promoting healthy gut bacteria.
    - *Dosage:* Start with a low dose and gradually increase, monitoring your tolerance over time. It's recommended to take prebiotics consistently for at least three weeks to assess their benefits.

11. **Low-FODMAP considerations**

    Many prebiotics, including inulin, are high-FODMAP and may trigger symptoms, making them tricky to incorporate during the elimination phase. Gentler prebiotics like PHGG and GOS may be more suitable. If you're following a low-FODMAP diet, introduce prebiotics gradually after the elimination phase, ideally with the guidance of a healthcare professional.

12. **Vitamin D**

    - *How it helps:* Supports gut health and immune function. Low vitamin D levels may worsen IBS symptoms.
    - *Dosage:* 1,000–2,000 IU daily, but consult a healthcare provider to assess your specific needs.

Note: Always consult with a healthcare provider before starting any new supplements, as they can interact with medications and might not be suitable for everyone based on their IBS type and overall health. Additionally, lifestyle changes like diet (such as the low FODMAP diet), stress management, and regular physical activity are also key to managing IBS effectively.

Tip #40: Choose Supplements Wisely and Track Your Reactions

Supplements such as probiotics or digestive enzymes can help support gut health, but not all supplements work for everyone. Start with small doses, track how your body responds, and introduce only one new supplement at a time to understand its effects. Consider keeping a journal to monitor any changes in symptoms.

***

My Personal Experience with Supplements

Supplements That Worked for Me:

1. **Turmeric (Curcumin)**: I take it with my evening meal, and it has always helped. Make sure it includes black pepper for better absorption.

2. **Magnesium**: Great for relieving constipation and improving sleep.

3. **Thiamine (Vitamin B1)**: This has helped with energy levels

and sleep. Be careful not to take too much though.

4. **Vitamin D**: I take this in the winter months. While it hasn't been a game-changer for IBS, it supports overall gut health and immunity.

5. **Probiotics**: I tried Bifidobacterium longum 35624, and it really seemed to help with bloating, abdominal pain and bowel movements. I would say try it for at least 6 weeks for it to take effect.

Supplements I Tried but Didn't Work:

1. **Peppermint Oil/Tea**: Instead of soothing my stomach, this actually aggravated my symptoms and gave me really bad heartburn that lasted a long time.

2. **Prebiotics**: I tried prebiotics a long time ago but don't remember the specific content (it was from Korea). I didn't see any noticeable health benefits. However, like I said, Inulin caused severe diarrhoea for me. I know that better-tolerated options like **partially hydrolysed guar gum** were recommended to me but I didn't follow through with it.

Supplements I Haven't Tried (But Are Recommended):

1. **Calcium Polycarbophil**: Helps normalise stool consistency for both IBS-C and IBS-D.

2. **Slippery Elm**: Coats and soothes the digestive tract.

3. **Digestive Enzymes**: Known to help break down food and reduce bloating.

4. **L-Glutamine**: Can support gut lining and reduce diarrhoea, especially in IBS-D cases.

When starting a supplement regime for IBS, it's essential to approach it with caution. Everyone's body responds differently, and factors like gut microbiome, stress levels, diet, and other health conditions play a significant role. Some people may experience relief from certain supplements, while others might see no benefit or even negative effects. Always start with small doses and monitor how your body reacts over time. It's wise to introduce only one new supplement at a time to gauge its effects accurately. If possible, consult a healthcare provider to ensure your safety.

***

Exercise and IBS: Finding What Works for Your Gut

Not long after I was diagnosed with IBS back in 2012, I figured getting back into exercise would be a surefire way to help manage my symptoms. I missed being active, so I decided to jump back into basketball, a sport I've always loved. One weekend, I found a local pick-up game in a small countryside town in Korea where I was living at the time. I was feeling pretty confident—thought I'd found the perfect solution to getting back on track.

Five minutes in, I was playing well, and everything seemed to be going great. "This is definitely the right decision," I thought to myself, feeling strong and energised. But then, about five minutes later, that all-too-familiar feeling hit me hard. I needed the toilet, and I needed it **badly**.

There were no bathrooms nearby, and suddenly, my panic set in. I apologised to the other players, bolted off the court, and ran through the town with a frantic desperation. I remember trying to open the doors of closed shops and restaurants, hoping one might be open. No luck. Eventually, I stumbled across a small restaurant with these old, fiery red doors—like fate, given my situation—where inside, workers were preparing mandu (Korean dumplings) for the day. It was still early morning, so there weren't any customers around—just confused workers watching a frantic foreigner shout, "Hwa-jang-sil" (Korean for toilet).

In their confusion, one of the workers pointed toward the back. I darted to the bathroom and finally found relief. The whole thing felt like it lasted an eternity, but afterwards, I had to make the humiliating walk back through the restaurant and leave. I didn't return to the courts that day—I just went home feeling embarrassed, wondering what had gone so terribly wrong.

This experience left me asking a lot of questions about IBS and exercise. I had assumed that getting active would help, but clearly, I hadn't thought things through enough.

What I Learned

That basketball game was a turning point for me. I realised that exercise could definitely help with my IBS, but I needed to be smarter about how I approached it. Here's what I learned from that experience:

- **Eat the Right Foods Before Exercise:** I hadn't thought about how my diet would play a role in that morning's game. Eating the wrong foods, especially IBS-trigger foods, before any exercise can lead to a disaster. It's essential to know your body and eat foods that will support your workout without causing an IBS flare-up.

- **Choose the Right Type of Exercise:** As much as I loved basketball, it's an intense sport with a lot of movement, which may not be the best choice when managing IBS. I needed to find exercises that were lower-impact but still effective—something like walking, tai chi or yoga to start.

- **Plan Ahead:** I should have known the area better and checked if there were any toilets nearby before playing. This is a key factor to avoid unnecessary stress during exercise, especially in unfamiliar places.

- **Mental Preparation is Key:** I realised that I had probably gone into the game with some underlying anxiety without even realising it. Worrying about my symptoms—whether consciously or not—was likely a trigger. Visualisation, meditation, and relaxation techniques beforehand (which we've covered in earlier chapters) could have helped calm my mind, preventing the situation from escalating.

So, I changed my approach. I swapped basketball for lower-impact activities like walking and Tai Chi. Eventually, I even took up table tennis, which is still active but much easier on my body. Over time, as my IBS became more manageable, I was able to return to basketball. It was a journey of trial and error, but I learned what my body needed to stay active without overwhelming my gut.

The Benefits of Exercise for IBS

Exercise can be a powerful tool in managing IBS symptoms, but like everything else, it's all about balance and finding what works for your body. Here's why exercise matters for IBS:

- **Improving Digestion:** Light to moderate exercise, such as walking or yoga, helps stimulate your digestive system. It can relieve constipation, reduce bloating, and improve gut motility, all of which are common IBS symptoms.
- **Reducing Stress:** Exercise releases endorphins, those "feel-good" hormones that help reduce stress and anxiety—key contributors to IBS flare-ups. Whether it's a calming yoga session or a walk in nature, physical activity can lower your body's stress response, making your gut feel more at ease.
- **Boosting Mental Health:** As we've covered earlier, the gut-brain connection plays a major role in IBS. Exercise can improve your overall mental health by reducing symptoms of anxiety and depression, creating a healthier environment for your gut. When your mind is calm, your digestive system often follows suit.

Choosing the Right Type of Exercise for IBS

Not all exercise is created equal when it comes to managing IBS. Some types of physical activity can improve symptoms, while others might exacerbate them. Here's a breakdown of different forms of exercise and how they affect IBS:

- **Low-Impact Exercises:** Activities like walking, swimming, Tai Chi, and yoga are generally great for those with IBS.

These exercises stimulate digestion, improve circulation, and reduce stress without overloading your body. They are gentle enough that you're less likely to experience an IBS flare-up.

- **High-Impact Exercises:** While high-intensity workouts like running, cycling, or HIIT (high-intensity interval training) can be great for overall fitness, they may not be suitable if you're prone to IBS symptoms. High-impact exercises can cause your body to release adrenaline and other stress hormones, which may worsen IBS symptoms like cramping or urgency. If you enjoy high-intensity workouts, start slow, track how your body responds, and make sure you've prepared well in terms of diet and stress management.

- **Core Strengthening & Pilates:** Strengthening your core can be particularly beneficial for digestion and overall gut health. Pilates, for example, is a low-impact workout that targets the muscles around your abdomen and pelvis, areas that play a key role in gut motility. Plus, these exercises focus on breathing, which can help calm the gut-brain axis.

- **Mind-Body Exercises:** Yoga, Tai Chi, and Qigong combine physical activity with mindfulness, breathing, and relaxation techniques. These practices can calm the nervous system and reduce stress—two factors that play a huge role in triggering IBS symptoms.

Ultimately, the best form of exercise for IBS is the one that works for your body without causing flare-ups. You may need to experiment to find the right balance, but low-impact, core-focused, and mind-body exercises are typically good places to start.

The Gut-Brain Axis and Exercise: Why They're Connected

As mentioned earlier, the gut-brain axis is a two-way communication system that links your brain and digestive system, influencing both your physical and mental well-being. Exercise can be a key factor in supporting this connection and alleviating IBS symptoms. Here's why:

- **Stress Reduction:** As we know, stress is a significant IBS trigger. Exercise helps lower cortisol and adrenaline levels, which can keep your gut from becoming overstimulated by stress signals.
- **Improved Circulation:** Exercise gets your blood flowing to all the right places, including your digestive system. Better circulation means smoother digestion and less chance of bloating or cramping.
- **Hormonal Balance:** Regular exercise helps balance hormones that influence both your mood and your gut. It boosts serotonin—the feel-good chemical that also keeps your digestion on track. And since most of your serotonin is made in the gut, it's yet another way your mind and gut are deeply connected.

By staying active, you're essentially "training" your gut to handle stress better and function more efficiently, creating a positive feedback loop that benefits both your mind and digestive health.

Tip #41: Make Exercise Your Gut's Best Friend

Exercise isn't just about keeping fit; it's a powerful ally in managing IBS when done right. Gentle, low-impact activities like walking, yoga, and Tai Chi can work wonders—they stimulate digestion, reduce stress, and strengthen the gut-brain connection without triggering symptoms. Think of every step, stretch, or mindful movement as a way to calm your mind and soothe your gut. Regular, balanced movement helps manage stress hormones, boosts mental clarity, and brings comfort to your digestion. Find activities that energise and uplift you, and make exercise a part of your wellness routine that supports your gut and whole-body health. Embrace movement as a long-term commitment to feeling better, one step at a time!

Practical Tips for Exercising with IBS

Staying active with IBS takes a bit of planning, but with the right approach, you can find what works best for your body. Here's how to make it easier:

- **Avoid Trigger Foods Pre-Workout:** What you eat before exercising matters. Steer clear of known trigger foods at least 2-3 hours before activity to avoid interruptions. Go for light, gut-friendly options like bananas, oatmeal, or rice cakes.

- **Stay Hydrated:** Dehydration can make IBS symptoms worse, so drink plenty of water before, during, and after your workout. Skip sugary sports drinks—they can irritate your gut.

- **Start Small and Gradually Increase Intensity:** If you're easing back into exercise, start with something simple, like a 10–15 minute walk. Gradually increase the intensity as your body gets used to it.

- **Listen to Your Body:** Pay close attention to how you feel. If a specific workout triggers symptoms, adjust your routine. Don't push through discomfort—finding the right balance is what matters most.

- **Plan Around Toilet Availability:** This is something I learned the hard way. If you're exercising in public or new areas, make sure you know where the nearest bathrooms are, just in case. This simple step can save you a lot of stress.

How to Incorporate Exercise into Your IBS Management Plan

Exercise works best when it's part of a well-rounded approach to managing IBS. Here's how to make physical activity fit seamlessly alongside other strategies like diet, relaxation, and mindfulness:

- **Pair Exercise with Relaxation:** After your workout, take a few minutes for mindfulness or deep breathing to calm your gut and reduce the chance of post-exercise flare-ups. This combo strengthens the gut-brain connection and helps you recover.

- **Make it a Habit:** Consistency is key. Start small by adding low-impact exercises like walking or yoga into your daily routine. Once you're comfortable, build up to longer or more frequent sessions—it's all about progress, not perfection.

- **Track What Works:** Keep a journal to log your symptoms, diet, and exercise habits. Over time, you'll spot patterns—like which workouts leave you feeling great and which ones might need tweaking.

Exercise can play an important role in managing your IBS, but like all things, it requires balance and mindfulness. With the right approach, exercise can improve not only your physical health but also help you take control of your symptoms and live a fuller, more active life.

Reflection and Practical Step

Medication and Supplements

When faced with the daily challenges of IBS, it's tempting to rely solely on medication for quick relief. But before reaching for that next pill, take a moment to pause and ask: Is this truly a long-term solution or just a temporary bandage? In this chapter, you've explored both traditional medications and natural supplements that can help manage symptoms. Let's take a moment to reflect on your current approach and take practical steps towards more mindful management.

Exercise: Reflection on Medication Use

Prompt:
Think about your current use of medication for IBS. Are there any medications you've come to rely on? How do you feel about this reliance, and are you open to gradually reducing your use while exploring other management options? Take time to reflect on the role medication plays in your IBS management, both physically and mentally.

Prompt 2:
Think about a time when you managed to reduce or delay your use of medication. What strategies did you use, and how did your body respond? Were there moments when you felt empowered or more in control? Reflect on what this experience taught you about balancing medication with other supportive practices.

Practical Step: Track Medication and Supplement Use

Start a medication and supplement diary. Each day, note what you take, why you take it, and how it affects your IBS symptoms. After a week, review the diary and see if you notice any patterns. Are there times when you reached for medication out of habit or anxiety rather than necessity? Use these insights to begin making more mindful decisions about how you manage your IBS with medication and supplements.

Practical Step: Set a SMART Goal for Exercise

Create a SMART (Specific, Measurable, Achievable, Relevant, Time-bound) goal for incorporating exercise into your IBS management plan. For example:

"I will go for a 20-minute walk three times a week for one month to see if it reduces my bloating and stress levels."

After the month, reflect on how the goal impacted your IBS symptoms. Did you notice improvements in digestion, mood, or energy? Adjust your next goal based on what worked well and what didn't. Setting clear, manageable goals allows you to build a sustainable exercise routine while paying attention to how your body responds. (More details on SMART goals are provided in Chapter 14, page 436)

Taking control of your medication, supplement use, and exercise routine is a powerful step toward long-term health management. By understanding when and why you turn to these tools, you create space to explore more holistic strategies, like mindful movement and relaxation techniques, that can bring lasting relief without reliance. Every small change—whether it's adjusting your medications, adding low-impact exercise, or simply tuning in to what your body needs—moves you closer to balance. Remember to be patient with yourself! With each mindful step, you're building a healthier, more confident version of yourself.

Chapter 14

The Long Game

Lifestyle Adjustments for IBS Relief

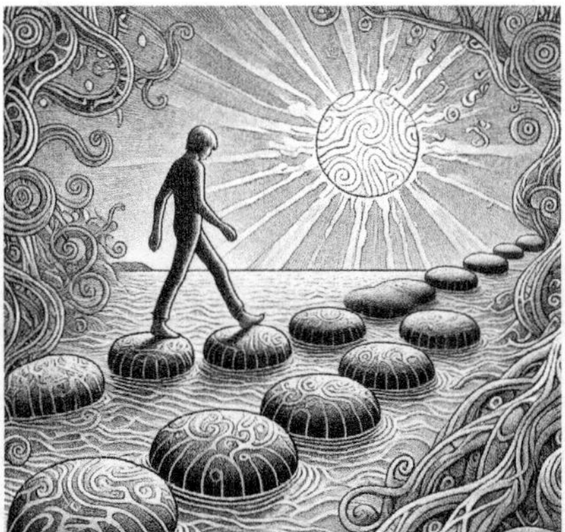

By now, you've journeyed through pages of practical tips, mindset shifts, and diet changes—all designed to help you navigate the choppy waters of living with IBS. But here's the thing: relief doesn't come from just one trick or a fleeting change. It comes from seeing the bigger picture, integrating these small adjustments into your life, and making a lasting commitment to your well-being.

When it comes to managing IBS, I've said it before, and I'll say it again because it's worth drilling in: unfortunately, this isn't about finding a "quick fix" or a band-aid solution that only offers temporary relief. I wish there was. Really. So think of everything you've learned so far—your mindful approach to stress, your understanding of trigger foods, the breathing techniques, and boundary-setting at work. These aren't just isolated pieces; they're interconnected parts of a whole. And that whole is the lifestyle you create for long-term relief. It's about the balance of your internal world—your thoughts, stress levels, and emotional health—with your external choices—what you eat, how you move, and the environment you shape around you.

The Goal: Sustainable Relief, Not Perfection

The goal here isn't to live perfectly or to be entirely free from symptoms all the time (wouldn't that be nice?), but to create a lifestyle that supports you in feeling your best most of the time. That's not all the time. Occasionally, I too may have flare-ups from time to time, but I reign it in and make sure I'm ticking the boxes of the things that I can actually control. So, this chapter will help you weave everything together, focusing on what long-term relief truly means: not just symptom management but creating a life that feels good, physically and emotionally.

Remember, "practice makes progress". It's definitely not about perfection here. If there's one thing you take away from this chapter, let it be this: IBS isn't something you "fix." It's something you manage and live alongside, creating a path that prioritises your well-being and allows you to move beyond the constraints of your symptoms.

Now, let's get to it and explore how you can integrate these tools into a lifestyle that not only eases your IBS but helps you thrive.

***

The Role of Mindset in Sustainable IBS Management

Adopting a Growth Mindset

A very long time ago, I read Dr. Carol Dweck's[1] book *Mindset*. It changed the way I viewed learning new things and how I approached progressing in my job, skills, and hobbies. If you are unaware, a growth mindset is a belief that challenges are opportunities for learning rather than obstacles—this is key. It's about shifting your focus to what you *can* do, rather than dwelling on what you can't. This journey is one of trial and error, and setbacks are bound to happen. But each setback isn't a failure; it's feedback. You might experience a flare-up despite your best efforts, or find that what worked for weeks suddenly isn't working anymore. Remember to be kind to yourself, and rather than throwing your hands up and declaring defeat, remind yourself that every bump in the road is a chance to understand your body better and make more informed choices.

---

1. Dr. Carol Dweck is a psychologist known for her research on mindset theory, introducing the "fixed" and "growth" mindsets. Her work shows that a growth mindset, viewing challenges as learning opportunities, fosters resilience and achievement.

As the great Marcus Aurelius[2] put it in his book *Meditations*, "*The impediment to action advances action. What stands in the way becomes the way.*" This quote captures the essence of turning challenges into opportunities. Rather than being discouraged by obstacles, Aurelius encourages us to see them as a path forward—something that shapes our intentions and actions. The very things that seem to block or hinder your progress can actually provide the guidance needed to adapt and move closer to your goal. So, when IBS symptoms flare up or setbacks occur, remember that they are not the end of the journey—they are the way through it.

Similarly, I think it's important to mention the Daoist concept of Wu-Wei, which I learned from the truly inimitably wonderful Alan Watts[3]. Wu-Wei or "effortless action," encourages us to move with the

---

2. Marcus Aurelius (121–180 AD) was a Roman Emperor and Stoic philosopher, best known for his work *Meditations*, a series of personal writings reflecting on duty, resilience, and self-discipline. His thoughts, grounded in Stoicism, emphasise virtue, wisdom, and maintaining composure in the face of adversity.

3. Alan Watts (1915–1973) was a British philosopher, writer, and speaker known for popularising Eastern philosophy, particularly Zen Buddhism and Taoism, in the Western world. Through his books and lectures, he explored the nature of existence, self-awareness, and the pursuit of harmony with the universe, blending humour and profound insight to inspire a deeper understanding of life and consciousness.

natural flow of life rather than resist it. For example, when you sail, you work with the wind, adjusting your sails to catch it properly. Trying to sail directly against the wind is futile, but if you adapt to its direction, you'll make progress effortlessly. So, it's about letting go of excessive control and aligning yourself with the rhythms of your body. This teaching really allowed me to embrace events as they come without forcing judgement or action, trusting that things will naturally play out. For IBS, this means not forcing change or getting overly anxious about every flare-up but instead adopting a calm acceptance. By doing so, you ease tension and respond more intuitively to your body's needs. Wu-Wei teaches that sometimes the best action is allowing things to be as they are, trusting that your body is capable of finding its balance when you're not fighting against it.

I would like to share my favourite Daoist story that embodies the concept of Wu-Wei completely and I have used and shared this story throughout my life and will continue to use it as inspiration for the ups and downs that my life will inevitably entail. I have heard this story in different variants, but this is how I know it as "Old Man White Horse":

Once upon a time, in a small village, there lived an old man, humble and wise, who owned a beautiful white horse. The villagers all admired this horse for its grace and strength, urging the old man to sell it for a fortune. But the old man refused, saying, "This horse is more than just a possession to me—it's a friend." One day, the horse ran away, vanishing into the wild, and the villagers mourned the man's loss, calling it a terrible misfortune. But the old man simply shrugged and said, "Maybe." Weeks later, the white horse returned, bringing with it a herd of wild horses. The villagers, wide-eyed with envy, congratulated the old man on his sudden luck. "What a blessing!" they exclaimed. But again, the old man was unfazed. "Maybe," he replied.

Shortly after, the old man's son tried to tame one of the wild horses but fell and broke his leg. The villagers gathered around, shaking their heads and clucking their tongues. "What a curse this horse has been! Now your only son is crippled." The old man, as calm as ever, said, "Maybe." A week later, war broke out in the region, and all able-bodied young men were drafted into the army. Many were sent off to fight and never returned. But the old man's son, with his broken leg, was spared from the battle. The villagers, astonished by the twists of fate, came to understand the old man's wisdom: nothing is inherently good or bad—it just is. And so, whenever something happened, the old man would smile and say, "Maybe," accepting life's changes without judgement, trusting in the flow of what comes and goes.

Managing IBS is a process of continual learning and self-discovery—one that requires patience, flexibility, and a bit of humour. Much like the old man with the white horse, your path won't be straightforward, and things won't always go the way you expect. And that's okay. Relief is not about finding a perfect, linear solution but about navigating the ups and downs with a sense of curiosity and openness.

As you journey through managing your IBS, remind yourself that it's about progress, not perfection. Every setback is simply another opportunity to learn more about your body and what it needs. And when you slip up, rather than beating yourself up, try to approach the situation as the old man would—with acceptance and grace. Ask,

"What can I learn from this?" and celebrate the small wins, whether it's finding a new food that doesn't trigger symptoms or successfully using a stress-relieving technique. Trust the process and know that, like any new habit, once you start celebrating those small victories, there's no looking back.

Tip #42: Listen to Your Body's Unique Signals
IBS management isn't a one-size-fits-all approach, and your body knows best. Pay attention to how it responds to different foods, routines, and habits. Trust yourself to make adjustments that feel right for you, and remember that your journey is unique.

Making Lasting Diet Changes

Personalising Your Diet

You've probably noticed that a one-size-fits-all approach doesn't work when it comes to diet and IBS. And that's a good thing! It means you have the freedom to explore and figure out what works best for you. The low FODMAP diet is a fantastic tool for identifying trigger foods, but it's meant to be the foundation, not a lifelong prescription. The real power comes in the reintroduction phase—where you test different foods and understand which ones you can enjoy without discomfort and which to steer clear from. Use this knowledge to build a diet that suits your needs, tastes, and lifestyle.

Ultimately, personalising your diet is about balance and flexibility. Know your "safe" foods, but allow yourself to be curious about new foods. Keeping a food diary can help you spot patterns, understand triggers, and adjust your diet to minimise symptoms while still enjoying your meals.

Tip #43: Embrace Flexibility Over Perfection

Remember, this journey isn't about getting everything perfect every day; it's about progress, patience, and showing up for yourself in small but powerful ways. Each step you take, whether it's committing to the restriction phase, building a new habit, or taking a moment to manage stress, all adds to strengthening your resilience. These efforts add up, even when they feel tough or tedious. Be proud of each positive choice, and trust that you're moving forward. Embrace the process, knowing that with each small step, you're creating a healthier, happier life. Keep going; you've got this!

Diet burnout is real, and sticking to a rigid eating plan forever isn't sustainable for most people. I resented my first 6 weeks of the low FODMAP diet massively. But after the restriction phase - that's where flexibility comes in. If it becomes too much, you can embrace the 80/20 rule: aim to make gut-friendly choices 80% of the time, but allow yourself to indulge a little without guilt. Life is too short to skip the occasional treat or favourite dish. The key is to enjoy those moments and move on, knowing you're making the best choices for your body most of the time.

Variety also plays a vital role. Eating the same thing every day—like chicken, broccoli, and rice—might seem like a safe option, but it can actually work against your recovery. A lack of variety can limit the nutrients your body needs to heal and thrive, and the reality is, it can get boring fast. When meals start feeling monotonous, it's easy to fall off track or turn to less helpful options.

Don't be afraid to experiment with new low-FODMAP recipes or mix up your meals to keep things fresh. Rotate ingredients, try seasonal fruits and vegetables, and get creative with herbs and spices to add flavour and excitement. When I was on the low-FODMAP diet, I stuck to a simple breakfast and a few variations for lunch, but I made it a point to experiment with dinner. It definitely made the process more enjoyable and effective.

Meal Planning and Preparation

Let's face it—nothing sets you up for success like being prepared. Meal planning isn't about spending hours in the kitchen every Sunday; it's about making life easier and ensuring you have nourishing options on hand. Here are some tips to support your diet for long-term relief:

- **Batch Cook**: A lot of you are probably used to this and know it well but by making large portions of safe meals and freezing them in single servings for nights when you just can't be bothered to cook are an absolute life-saver. Things I made a lot were shepherd's pie, chicken curry and a low-FODMAP version of a beef chilli con carne – basically switching beans for lentils.

- **Stock Up on Low-FODMAP Snacks**: Keep a stash of easy-to-grab snacks like rice cakes, lactose-free yoghurts, or homemade energy bars so you're never caught off-guard when hunger hits. Please see the list of snacks in the food section of the low-FODMAP diet.

- **Maintain a "Safe" Foods Grocery List**: Keep a running list of your go-to low-FODMAP foods. When it's time to shop, you'll know exactly what to buy and won't waste time figuring out what you need. I remember my first time trying to buy food for the week during the restriction phase of the low FODMAP diet, and I swear I was in the supermarket for nearly three hours!! So remember to plan ahead.

At the end of the day, the goal is to make eating well as effortless as possible. The easier it is to stick to your personalised diet, the more likely it will become a sustainable part of your lifestyle—and that's when the magic happens. By planning ahead, you're not just preparing meals; you're setting yourself up for long-term relief and success.

***

Stress Management as a Lifestyle

Daily Habits for Reducing Stress

Managing stress, especially when it comes to IBS, is a marathon—not a sprint. Throughout this book, you've come across a variety of techniques designed to help reduce stress: mindfulness, breathing exercises, journaling, and more. But having the tools isn't enough; integrating these habits into your daily routine is what will truly make a difference. And to make these habits stick, we need to talk about one key thing: how to build and maintain habits effectively.

The Habit Loop

In 2012, I came across the book *The Power of Habit by* Charles Duhigg. I was trying to create a language-learning routine but was unable to make it stick. What I learned from the book was that to build a habit that lasts, it's crucial to understand the "Habit Loop". Once I learned this I was able to implement so many new habits in my life. The loop consists of three simple steps:

1. **Cue**: The trigger that initiates the habit. For example, feeling stressed could be the cue to practise a breathing exercise.

2. **Routine**: The action itself—the habit you're trying to build. In this case, that could be your breathing routine or a mindful meditation practice.

3. **Reward**: The positive reinforcement you receive from completing the habit, such as the feeling of calmness or relief from IBS symptoms.

By understanding and intentionally creating this loop, you can reinforce habits that promote long-term stress relief. Here's how you can do that for IBS management:

- **Find a Cue**: Tie your new habit to an existing routine or behaviour. For instance, if you want to start a morning breathing practice, link it to an existing cue like brushing your teeth. Every time you brush your teeth, it becomes a reminder to spend 2 minutes doing deep breathing. If journaling is your focus, use winding down for bed as your cue.

- **Choose the Routine**: Make it simple and achievable. If you try to meditate for 30 minutes from day one, it can feel like too big a commitment, making you less likely to follow through. Instead, start with a 5-minute session of guided meditation using an app like *Headspace* or *Calm*. The key is to make it so easy that it's hard not to do it. Over time, you can build on that foundation and lengthen your practice as it becomes part of your routine.

- **Reward Yourself**: Find an immediate reward that reinforces the habit. For example, after a breathing session, you might reward yourself with a cup of herbal tea, a walk, some dark chocolate or your favourite playlist. Over time, the act itself will become the reward as you start to experience less stress and improved IBS symptoms, but giving yourself that initial boost can help make the habit stick.

The Power of Tiny Gains - The 1% Rule

When I was at my lowest point with IBS, the idea of getting better felt impossible. I wanted quick results—some magic pill that would fix everything. But that's not how it works, is it? If you're reading this, you've probably already figured out that real, lasting change doesn't come overnight. It comes from consistency. In one of my jobs, a colleague of mine would occasionally give me motivational post-it notes from a book that would later become instrumental to overcoming other areas of my life, but it is 100% relevant to overcoming IBS. In his book *Atomic Habits*, James Clear talks about the idea of getting just 1% better every day. At first, it sounds almost laughable—what difference could 1% possibly make? But when you add it up over time, those tiny improvements create real, lasting change. It's the power of compounding, and the truth is that small steps matter more than we think.

There's an old story I read as a child that fits perfectly to this. It's about a king who was tricked into giving away his rice supply in what seemed like a harmless bet. The king was asked to place a single grain of rice on the first square of a chessboard and then double the amount on each subsequent square. It didn't seem like much—a grain here, a grain there. But by the time he reached the 64th square, the amount of rice required was astronomical, far more than the king could ever have imagined. The king, like many of us, didn't realise the power of compounding. What starts as something small can quickly grow into something much larger, and this principle applies just as much to our health and habits as it does to grains of rice.

When it comes to managing IBS, this concept makes all the difference. You don't have to overhaul your entire life all at once. You just have to focus on making small, manageable changes every day. Whether it's learning a new stress management technique, tweaking your diet, or working on your mindset, every little step counts. Trust me, the results will come.

The Science Behind Small Changes

Think of it like this: if you improve by just 1% every day, by the end of the year, you're 37% better than where you started. It doesn't sound like much, but it adds up. This is exactly how you can approach managing your IBS.

You don't need to fix everything overnight. Start by making a small adjustment to your routine— Maybe try practising rhythmic breathing for just five minutes or take a moment to reframe a negative thought before it spirals into stress. These tiny changes, when done consistently, have a ripple effect. Your gut starts to calm, your stress levels lower, and slowly but surely, you start to notice real progress.

The beauty of this approach is that it removes the pressure. You don't have to be perfect. You just have to keep moving forward, one small step at a time.

Tip #44: Embrace Patience and Persistence

Lasting changes don't happen overnight. IBS management is about building habits that support you over time. Be patient with yourself, celebrate small wins, and keep going. Every small step you take is moving you closer to better health and resilience.

The Mindset Shift: Focus on Progress, Not Perfection

Here's the part where I tell you something I wish I'd known from the start: you don't have to be perfect to make progress. When you're dealing with IBS, it's easy to feel like you're constantly messing up—whether it's slipping on your diet, missing a stress management practice, or just having a bad day. But the truth is, none of us are perfect. The goal isn't perfection—it's progress.

This is where the 1% improvement mindset really shines. You don't need to get everything right all the time. You just need to focus on getting a little better every day. Maybe your IBS symptoms flared up today—that's okay. What's one thing you can do tomorrow that might help? That's what matters: those small, steady steps forward. They're the ones that last.

Reflection

Building Resilience Through Small Changes

When I look back at my journey, it wasn't the big, dramatic changes that made the difference—it was the small, everyday improvements. At first, it didn't feel like much. But over time, I started to notice fewer flare-ups, less anxiety, and better control over my symptoms. It wasn't overnight, and it wasn't easy, but it was worth it.

For anyone out there struggling with IBS, my advice is this: don't get overwhelmed by the thought of having to change everything at once. Focus on those 1% improvements. Every time you make a small change—whether it's what you eat, how you manage stress, or how you take care of your body—you're moving forward. And over time, those tiny improvements add up to big, lasting changes.

Here's the challenge: think of one small thing you can do today that will get you 1% closer to where you want to be. Maybe it's practising deep breathing for five minutes. Maybe it's swapping one meal for a low-FODMAP option. Or maybe it's simply taking a moment to reframe your mindset when the anxiety kicks in.

Whatever it is, start small, and don't worry about doing everything perfectly. Just focus on that 1% improvement. Because in the end, it's not about how fast you move—it's about the direction you're heading. And if you keep moving forward, even by just 1%, you'll be amazed at how far you can go. Below are some examples of what you can do now to make these small changes:

- **Breathing**: Start with just one minute of rhythmic breathing, focusing on a longer exhale than inhale. This is easy to incorporate and immediately calming, setting the tone for your day.
- **Progressive Muscle Relaxation**: Spend a couple of minutes each day tensing and then relaxing different muscle groups, starting from your toes and working up to your head. This helps bring awareness to areas of tension and encourages physical relaxation.
- **Visualisation Practice**: Take a minute each morning to close your eyes and visualise a calming place or a moment of peace. Imagine the sights, sounds, and sensations of that place to set a calm tone for your day.
- **Walking Breaks**: If you're feeling stuck or anxious, take a brief one-minute walk around your home, office, or outside. This quick movement can help clear your mind and relieve stress.

- **Journaling**: Don't aim to write pages—begin with a short gratitude entry. One to three lines about what you're thankful for can shift your focus away from stress and create a habit of positivity.

Environment Design: Setting Yourself Up for Success

Another concept from *Atomic Habits* is "environment design"—essentially, shaping your environment so that it encourages positive habits and discourages bad ones. Think of this as creating an atmosphere that supports your stress-management goals:

- **Visible Reminders**: Leave a journal on your nightstand so that you're reminded to write before bed. Place a yoga mat in your living room so it's easy to start your stretching routine.

- **Avoiding Temptation**: If certain activities increase stress (like checking work emails late at night), create physical barriers to avoid them. For instance, keep your phone out of the bedroom to discourage screen time before sleep.

- **Habit Stacking**: Similar to the ideas in *the power of habit,* link a new habit to an existing one. For example, if you drink tea every evening, use that as a cue to practise a 5-minute deep breathing session while waiting for the tea to brew.

Make It Social: Accountability and Support

One of the most effective ways to build a lasting habit is by getting others involved. Social accountability can be a powerful motivator:

- **Join a Group or Challenge**: If you're aiming to incorporate more movement into your day, consider joining a local walking group or participating in a virtual yoga class. Personally, I engage in Tai Chi both online and offline. Additionally, IBS support groups—both online and in-person—can be invaluable. They offer a safe space to share experiences, learn coping strategies, and connect with others who understand your journey.

For example:

- In the UK, explore support groups through The IBS Network.

The IBS Network

- Online communities such as the IBS Patient Support Group, the IBS Group Forum, or the Inspire IBS Support Community are accessible to everyone, regardless of location.

IBS Patient Support Group

the IBS Group Forum

Inspire IBS Support Community

These communities offer a chance to connect with like-minded individuals, swap stories, discover practical tips, and find the kind of support that makes managing IBS feel a little less overwhelming.

- **Share Your Goals with a Friend**: Let someone close to you know about your commitment to managing your IBS through these new habits. It could be as simple as sending a quick message each day about what stress-reducing activity you did. I am fortunate enough to have a wonderful wife who supports me and reminds me of the things I am committed to doing.
- **Create a Habit Tracker**: This can be as simple as a calendar on the fridge or a checklist in your planner. Marking off each day you complete your habit can provide a visual cue for your progress and keep you motivated.

Design for Consistency, Not Perfection

I feel like I've been repeating myself endlessly here, but it's important. Remember, the goal is not to do everything perfectly. There will be days when you don't get to practise mindfulness, skip a breathing exercise, or forget to write in your journal. That's okay! What matters is that you get back to your habits without guilt or self-judgement. Consistency over time will bring more benefits than striving for perfection and burning out.

When these small habits become part of your daily routine, they add up to create a more stress-resilient lifestyle. Your body and mind become more capable of managing the stressors that come with IBS, allowing you to respond to flare-ups and stress in a calm, balanced way.

By integrating these practices into your life one small step at a time, you're not just creating habits—you're creating a lifestyle that supports both your emotional well-being and your gut health. Remember: progress over perfection, one mindful moment at a time.

Movement and Exercise for Your Gut and Mind

Exercise, when done in a way that's enjoyable, can significantly improve your stress levels and overall well-being. And don't forget—your gut health benefits from movement too.

Gentle, IBS-friendly exercises include:

- **Walking**: One of the simplest yet most effective ways to stay active. Whether it's a morning stroll or a quick walk during your lunch break, the important thing is to move. I'm a big fan of this as I've gotten older. I just love an hour or two of walking in the countryside.
- **Yoga**: Yoga is an amazing way to stretch, strengthen, and de-stress without overloading your digestive system. Try gentle forms like yin or hatha yoga, which focus on mindful breathing and relaxation. Despite trying out yoga, I found it wasn't for me (and that's ok!).
- **Stretching and Low-Impact Exercises**: Not all movement has to break a sweat. Stretching in the morning or after a long day at work can help ease tension and reduce stress.

The main takeaway here is to find what feels good for you and stick to it. Consistency is more important than intensity, and when you find an activity you enjoy, you're more likely to keep it as part of your long-term routine.

Work-Life Balance and Setting Boundaries

Stress doesn't just come from big life changes or overwhelming situations—it's often the small, cumulative stressors from work and everyday life that build up. Remember the work stress chapter? It all boils down to setting boundaries and reclaiming your space.

Learning to say "no" confidently was a big turning point for me, and it can be for you too. It's not about being rude or dismissive; it's about prioritising your health. Setting boundaries at work, both physically and mentally, is just so important. If possible, create an "off-time" from work emails and devices, allowing space for yourself to unwind without the constant buzz of notifications. Small changes, like scheduling regular breaks throughout your workday or ensuring you leave work at a reasonable hour, can go a long way in maintaining a balanced and less stressful lifestyle.

***

Cultivating Healthy Sleep Habits

As we all know, good sleep is the bedrock of a healthy lifestyle—without it, even the best stress management strategies and diet adjustments can fall short. Revisit the sleep habits discussed previously: sticking to a consistent sleep schedule (yes, that means weekends too!), limiting caffeine and alcohol before bed, creating a calm wind-down routine, and setting up a restful sleep environment. The goal is to create a sleep pattern that supports both your mind and body, allowing you to reset and wake up ready to tackle whatever comes your way.

To optimise your sleep, consider your environment. Think of your room as a sanctuary—keep it dark, cool, and quiet. If necessary, invest in items like blackout curtains, an eye mask, a good-quality mattress, and earplugs to support an environment conducive to restful sleep. Sleep plays such a significant role in managing your IBS symptoms and your stress levels that any effort you make to improve it is time well spent.

Troubleshooting Sleep Issues: When Things Aren't Quite Right

For some, despite best efforts, sleep remains elusive. And that's okay—it's about trying different strategies until you find what works. If you find yourself struggling, here are some additional tips:

- **Natural Supplements**: Magnesium can help calm the nervous system and promote better sleep. Chamomile tea, sipped about an hour before bed, is a classic for a reason—it has gentle, calming effects that can ease you into rest.

- **L-theanine**, known for its relaxing properties, and **ashwagandha**, which helps manage stress, are also worth exploring.

- **Using Melatonin**: Melatonin can be a useful tool for adjusting your sleep-wake cycle, especially for falling asleep faster. But from my experience, it's important to use it cautiously. Over time, I found I needed higher doses, and eventually, I couldn't sleep without it. Use it sparingly and consult with your healthcare provider to avoid dependency.

- **Speaking with a Professional**: Don't hesitate to reach out to a sleep specialist, counsellor, or doctor for guidance if sleep issues persist. Chronic sleep problems can significantly impact your quality of life, so seeking professional support can be a life-changing move. I did this and was on supplements and melatonin for around 6 months when I was in a bad place with regard to sleep.

***

Physical Environment and Space for Relaxation

Creating a Relaxing Home Environment

Your home should be a place of peace and relaxation—a buffer from the stressors of the outside world. An organised, peaceful living space can play a huge role in your overall well-being. I am naturally a messy, disorganised person. There. I said it. But I have thrown stuff out and tried to live a more minimalist life. As you can imagine, decluttering can help clear your mental space as much as your physical one. You don't need to transform your home into a minimalist haven, but making small changes like having a tidy desk, keeping your bedroom clear of excess items, and adding a few plants or candles can make a difference in how relaxed you feel in your space.

Hobbies and Passion Projects as Stress-Relief Tools

Hobbies aren't just about filling time—they're about filling your life with activities that bring you joy and relaxation. Dedicate time to activities that help you decompress, whether it's a creative outlet like painting, crocheting (my wife is a huge fan), or even listening to your favourite music. Hobbies allow your mind to shift focus away from daily stressors and onto something enjoyable. Not only does this help break up your day, but it also allows your mind to unwind and recalibrate.

Find something you genuinely enjoy and make time for it regularly. Start something new too. I didn't know I liked gardening until I started to help out on the family allotment. All of a sudden, I'm growing every vegetable I can think of! Whether it's photography, dancing, or even learning a new skill—these activities can be therapeutic and help reset your mind. The idea is to fill your life with moments of joy that serve as breaks from stress, making it easier to manage your IBS in the long run.

Social Connections and Support Systems

Cultivating Supportive Relationships

It's no secret—living with IBS can sometimes make you feel isolated. But you don't have to do this alone. Relationships—whether with friends, family, or a supportive community—are so important for emotional well-being and resilience. Having people you trust and who understand your situation can make all the difference. Share your IBS journey with those who care about you. I'm not saying you need to broadcast your symptoms to everyone, but letting a few key people know what you're going through can provide that emotional buffer when times get tough. Knowing that someone "gets it" can definitely alleviate stress and anxiety, and allow you to open up when you need support.

Seeking Professional Help

There's also no shame in reaching out for professional guidance. Think of it as building your "IBS management team." This can include counsellors for stress management, dietitians for nutritional needs, or medical professionals for tailored treatment options. I'm not afraid to say I've seen therapists, done online courses on overcoming anxiety, and been on specific diet plans, among other things. Getting help isn't a sign of weakness—it's a sign of strength and self-care. Taking that step to speak to someone who can help you navigate your mental and physical health needs is not only proactive, but it's a long-term investment in yourself.

***

Setting Goals for IBS Management

Having goals can make the journey of IBS management more structured and less overwhelming. But the key is to set small, specific, and realistic goals that work for your lifestyle. I can't stress this enough: it's very easy to make these big, elaborate goals, only to fall short, feel tremendous guilt, and self-hatred, and give up, leading to anxiety and inaction. The cycle continues, and nothing gets done. So, please make sure that it is, in fact, a SMART goal.

For example, maybe your long-term goal is to reduce stress and manage flare-ups effectively, but your short-term goal could be to practise a five-minute breathing exercise daily or eliminate a trigger food for one month. The idea is to have a target that's not only achievable but also meaningful to you—something you know will have a direct impact on how you feel.

Why SMART Goals Matter

Setting SMART goals helps clarify your path, keeps you motivated, and increases your chances of success. When you break down what each element of SMART means, it becomes clear why this approach is so effective:

- **Specific**: Your goal should be clear and detailed. Instead of saying, "I want to manage my stress better," be specific: "I will practise a five-minute breathing exercise each morning."

- **Measurable**: You need a way to track your progress. For example, if your goal is to add stress management techniques, measure it by aiming for "three five-minute breathing sessions a week" to assess if you're on track.

- **Achievable**: Make sure your goal is realistic within your current constraints. Aiming to meditate for an hour daily might be too ambitious initially. Start with five minutes and increase gradually.

- **Relevant**: Ensure the goal aligns with your larger objectives. For IBS management, this might mean focusing on practices that directly impact your symptoms, such as dietary changes or stress reduction.
- **Time-bound**: Set a deadline or timeframe to give yourself structure and motivation. "I will try eliminating a specific trigger food for one month and then evaluate my symptoms."

Examples of SMART Goals for IBS Management

To give you some inspiration, here are a bunch of practical examples of SMART goals:

- "I will go for a 20-minute walk in the park every morning, five days a week, for the next month."
- "I'll practise progressive muscle relaxation for 10 minutes before bed three times a week for the next month."
- "I will swap my evening drink with a chamomile tea and track my sleep quality for two weeks."
- "I will introduce one new low-FODMAP vegetable each week and keep a food journal to note any changes over a month."
- "I'll practise rhythmic breathing for three minutes before

each meal, five days a week, for the next month."

- "I will spend 15 minutes journaling three nights a week to reflect on my stress levels and identify triggers over the next month."
- "I will attend a yoga class twice a week for the next six weeks to improve relaxation and physical well-being."
- "I'll schedule 10 minutes of visualisation practice in the morning, four days a week, for the next three weeks."
- "I will practise mindful eating by setting aside time to eat without distractions for lunch every day, five days a week, for the next month."

Tips for Staying on Track

1. Reflect and Adjust: Regularly reflect on your progress. If a goal feels too challenging or isn't working, adjust it. Flexibility is key to sustaining long-term habits.
2. Celebrate Small Wins: Acknowledge and celebrate when you meet a goal, no matter how small. This reinforces positive behaviour and keeps you motivated.
3. Stay Accountable: Share your goals with a friend or keep a journal to track your progress and hold yourself accountable.

Setting goals in this way gives you direction, helps you manage IBS step by step, and empowers you to make lasting, meaningful changes without feeling overwhelmed. Remember, each small step counts and contributes to your overall well-being.

Tracking Progress and Celebrating Wins

Monitoring your progress isn't just about spotting patterns or triggers; it's about celebrating the wins—both big and small. Keep a journal to record what's working, what's not, and what you've learned along the way. Did you make it through a week without a flare-up? Amazing—celebrate that win. Managed to stick to your sleep schedule? Pat yourself on the back! By tracking progress and recognising achievements, you maintain motivation and see tangible results from your efforts.

***

Dealing with Setbacks

Flare-ups are going to happen. 100%. Without fail. And let me tell you—it's easy to feel defeated when they do. Not just defeated but depressed, angry, lonely and helpless. But rather than spiralling into panic mode or frustration, remind yourself that setbacks are part of the journey. Your goal is not to eliminate all symptoms forever, but to manage them in a way that lets you live comfortably and happily. Use flare-ups as an opportunity to revisit what's working and what needs adjusting. Is your stress creeping back up? Is a new food affecting you? Take a deep breath, reflect, and move forward. Treat flare-ups like data points that help refine your approach rather than catastrophes that derail your progress.

Crafting Your Ideal Routine

By now, you have a whole toolkit of strategies for managing your IBS—from diet and exercise to stress reduction and sleep habits. The next step is to integrate these elements into a routine that feels natural and sustainable for you. Start with the basics and build on them:

- **Morning Routine**: Begin your day with a gentle stretch, mindful breathing, or a short walk to set a positive tone.
- **Balanced Meals**: Plan meals and snacks throughout the day, focusing on low-FODMAP choices that support your gut health.
- **Midday Breaks for Mindfulness**: Take a pause in your day to reset—whether it's a quick breathing exercise, mindful eating during lunch, or a short walk.
- **Evening Wind-Down**: Use evenings to disconnect from work, practise a relaxing activity, and prepare for restful sleep.

You don't need to follow a rigid schedule—think of these as rhythms to shape your day. Over time, they become second nature, contributing to long-term relief and well-being.

Making Adjustments Along the Way

Life is unpredictable, and what works today might need tweaking tomorrow. The important thing is to be adaptable and willing to make changes as needed. If you find that a certain habit isn't working, try something else. If your routine feels too overwhelming, strip it back to the essentials. The key is to be flexible and keep an open mind, understanding that your needs may shift over time, and that's okay.

Tip #45: Be Kind to Yourself

IBS management can be challenging, and it's easy to be hard on yourself. Remember that self-compassion is part of healing. Recognise your efforts, acknowledge your challenges, and treat yourself with the same kindness you'd offer a friend on a similar journey.

Conclusion

Living Well with IBS

Managing IBS is about creating harmony between your internal and external worlds. It's about cultivating a mindset that embraces learning and growth, establishing a diet that supports your gut, developing habits that alleviate stress, and shaping an environment that promotes relaxation. When these elements come together, they work in harmony to provide long-term relief and make life more manageable and enjoyable.

Encouragement and Practicality

You've made it through this chapter, and hopefully, the entire book—so congratulations! This is no small feat. Know that taking control of your health is an empowering journey, and the small steps you take every day will add up to significant improvements over time. Be patient with yourself. Change doesn't happen overnight, and that's okay. Use reminders, track your progress, and above all, celebrate every step forward.

Now it's your turn. Don't just close this book and go back to your usual routine. Take what you've learned and put it into action. Try one of the breathing exercises, start a food diary, get out for a walk, or set a reminder for worry time. Remember, every small effort is progress toward a healthier, happier life. You have the tools, the knowledge, and the mindset. Now, it's time to go out there and create the life you deserve.

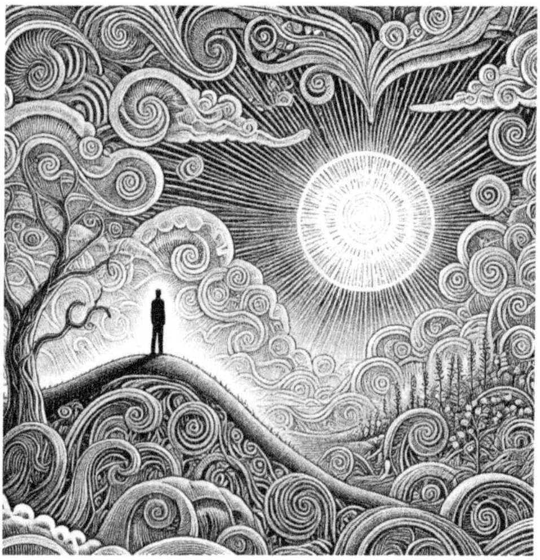

Checklist for Practical Steps

I would like to take a moment to reflect on all the practical steps you've worked through. Below is a checklist of all the practical steps covered throughout the book. Use this to track your progress, and to revisit any strategies you may want to try again or continue practising.

Chapter 1: IBS in Society

- **Start a Symptom Diary**: For the next week, note down what you eat, your stress levels, and how your gut responds throughout the day. Try to include emotional responses as well. This diary can help you start identifying patterns between your food, stress, and symptoms.

Chapter 2: The Mind-Body Connection

- **Practise Worry Time**: Dedicate 20 minutes daily to address anxious thoughts. Write them down throughout the day and process them during this window. Let go of worries until the next session.

- **Apply the 2-Minute Rumination Rule**: Limit rumination to 2 minutes using a timer. Reflect briefly on whether it helped or taught you anything, then let it go to regain focus and clarity.

Chapter 3: Breaking the Vicious Cycle

- **Meditation**: Practise meditating for 5–10 minutes daily. Find a quiet spot, focus on your breath, and relax. Pair it with a routine, like after your morning tea.
- **Rhythmic Breathing**: Try 7/11 breathing—inhale for 7 seconds and exhale for 11. Adjust the ratio to what feels natural. Practise during breaks or before meals to manage stress.
- **Affirmations**: During meditation or breathing exercises, repeat affirmations like "My gut is calm." Use them 2–3 times daily to reinforce a sense of control.
- **Visualisation**: Imagine a calming scene during moments of stress. Engage all your senses to create a vivid, relaxing mental picture.
- **Forest Bathing**: Spend time in nature once a week. Focus on the sights and sounds around you to calm your mind and body.

- **Autogenic Relaxation**: Follow a guided video to learn this technique, then practise independently. Focus on sensations of warmth and relaxation in your body once or twice daily.

Chapter 4: From Chaos to Calm: Tackling Internal Stress

- **Progressive Muscle Relaxation (PMR)**: Practise PMR once this week, especially before bed or during high stress. Focus on relaxing each part of your body to release tension and calm your nervous system.
- **Belly Breathing**: Spend 5–10 minutes practising belly breathing daily. Use it during moments of anxiety to activate your body's relaxation response and soothe your gut.
- **Reframe Stressful Situations:** Ask yourself, "What can I control right now?" or "How can I respond differently?" Shifting your perspective reduces overwhelm and fosters a sense of empowerment.
- **Set Emotional Boundaries:** Visualise a protective bubble or glass wall to keep negativity out while allowing positive engagement with others.
- **Develop Self-Compassion:** Replace self-criticism with kindness. Remind yourself that you're doing your best, just as you would reassure a friend.
- **Practise Mindfulness and Grounding:** Use grounding

exercises like rhythmic breathing or observing your surroundings to stay present and centred during stress.

- **Use the STOP Method:** Stop what you're doing, take a deep breath, observe your feelings without judgement, and proceed mindfully with a deliberate response.
- **Practise Emotional Regulation:** Recognise stress as it builds. Acknowledge your emotions and use a calming technique like belly breathing or grounding to regain control and prevent escalation.

Chapter 5: Emotional Triggers

- **Emotion Check-in**: Spend 3 minutes each day pausing to name your emotions without judgement. This simple practice builds self-awareness, helping you recognise feelings before they impact your body.
- **Practise RAIN**: When a strong emotion arises, recognise it, allow it to be there, investigate how it feels in your body, and nurture yourself with kindness, as you would a friend.
- **Visualise Emotions as Waves**: Imagine emotions as waves rising, peaking, and falling. This visualisation reminds you that emotions are temporary and helps you stay calm during intense moments.
- **Weekly Letting Go Exercise**: At the end of the week, visualise releasing a stressful emotion. Picture it drifting away,

like a cloud, while taking a deep breath to reinforce emotional closure.

Chapter 6: The Power of Your Mind's Eye: Healing IBS Through Imagery

- **Combine Techniques for Stress Management**: This week, pair visualisation with grounding or rhythmic breathing. For example, while using the future history method, start with grounding exercises or 7/11 breathing. This combination reinforces calmness and prepares you mentally and physically for future events.

Chapter 7: Outside In: How External Stressors Fuel IBS

No Practical Steps

Chapter 8: Balancing External Demands: Stress Management Beyond the Self

- **Time Management with the Pomodoro Technique**: Use the Pomodoro Technique for one day by working in 25-minute intervals with 5-minute breaks. After four sessions, take a 15–30 minute break. Reflect on how this structure impacts your focus, productivity, and stress.

- **Redefine Success from Perfection to Progress**: Pick one task to complete with the aim of "good enough" instead of perfection. Set a time limit, finish the task, and move on. Notice how this shift affects your stress levels and overall mindset.

Chapter 9: Bonds and Boundaries: How Relationships Shape Your Gut Health

- **Evaluate Your Relationships**: Use the relationship evaluation questionnaire from earlier in the chapter to assess how your relationships influence your stress and IBS symptoms. Answer honestly and use the insights to guide any needed changes.
- **Set Boundaries with Toxic Individuals**: Identify one stressful relationship and set a clear boundary this week, such as limiting contact or having an honest conversation. Observe how this affects your emotional well-being and IBS symptoms.

Chapter 10: Managing Work Stress: Finding Balance in a Busy World

- **Set One Work Boundary This Week**: Choose one work boundary, such as leaving at a set time or avoiding emails after hours, and stick to it. Reflect on how this impacts your stress levels and overall well-being.
- **Take a Mindful Micro-Break**: Schedule 3–5 minute breaks for breathing exercises or stretching during your

workday. Notice how these moments of calm affect your stress and IBS symptoms.

- **Practise the Two-Minute Rule**: Complete tasks that take less than two minutes right away. This reduces the buildup of small tasks, easing stress and mental clutter.

- **Reflect on Your "Why"**: Spend time journaling about the purpose behind your work beyond earning a paycheck. Reconnecting with your "why" can help reduce burnout and make work feel more meaningful.

Chapter 11: Rest and Digest: How Sleep Heals Your Gut

- **Set a Consistent Sleep Schedule:** Commit to going to bed and waking up at the same time every day, including weekends. Track how this consistency impacts both your sleep quality and IBS symptoms over the week.

- **Create a Relaxing Wind-Down Routine:** Implement a calming pre-sleep routine for at least 30 minutes before bed. Whether it's reading, stretching, or listening to soothing music, choose an activity that signals to your body that it's time to relax and prepare for rest.

- **Limit Stimulants and Adjust Evening Habits:** Pay attention to your caffeine and alcohol intake. Try cutting off caffeine by early afternoon and avoid alcohol in the evenings. Also, avoid large meals right before bed, giving your body time to digest and relax before sleeping.

- **Optimise Your Sleep Environment:** Ensure that your bedroom is cool, dark, and quiet. Consider using earplugs, an eye mask, or blackout curtains if needed to create a sleep-friendly atmosphere that helps you fall and stay asleep more easily.

Chapter 12: From Plate to Peace: Mindful Eating and Gut-Friendly Nutrition

- **Commit to the Low-FODMAP Diet**: Take the first step this week by fully committing to the low-FODMAP diet. Focus on consistency to gain insights into your food triggers. Embrace the process one day at a time, and remember that every effort brings you closer to lasting symptom relief and better control over your gut health.

- **Take Control, One Small Change at a Time**: Start reducing or eliminating alcohol and coffee from your routine. Swap an alcoholic drink for a mocktail or your morning coffee for herbal tea. If ready, commit to a week or more without these triggers, track your symptoms, and notice improvements in gut health, mood, and energy.

Chapter 13: Medications, Supplements, and the Role of Exercise in IBS Management

- **Track Medication and Supplement Use**: Start a diary to

log what medication and supplements you take, why you take them, and how they affect your IBS symptoms. After a week, review for patterns and reflect on whether you're using them mindfully or out of habit. Use this insight to make more informed decisions about your management plan.

- **Set a SMART Goal for Exercise**: Create a SMART goal to integrate exercise into your IBS routine. For example: "I will walk for 20 minutes three times a week for one month to reduce bloating and stress." Reflect after the month on how it impacted your symptoms and adjust your goal as needed to build a sustainable routine.

Epilogue

So, to the question you were all asking yourselves at the start—did I end up shitting myself roadside on a motorway in Seoul, South Korea?

The simple answer, thankfully, is no, though my bowels felt as if they were auditioning for a disaster movie. While I'm sure my dramatic dash off the bus, yelling about death and hospitals, lives on in the memory of some bewildered commuter, the story didn't end in total calamity.

After the bus pulled away and left me standing by the side of the road, I paced anxiously, scanning the South Korean motorway for any semblance of privacy—a bush, a tree, even an implausibly appearing public toilet. The sweat poured down my face as my gut twisted in revolt. In that moment, a single thought cut through the chaos: Walk. Just walk and breathe. With each step and a few deep, deliberate breaths, luckily, the relentless urgency began to ease as if my body had decided to grant me a rare moment of mercy.

After what felt like hours, a building appeared in the distance, and I made a beeline for it. Yet, I tempered my hope—a cautious trick I'd learned—knowing the feeling of needing the toilet intensifies with expectations. Also, many buildings in Korea have keypads on restroom doors, and I prepared myself for disappointment. But fortune smiled on me that day: the door was unlocked, and relief was finally, blessedly mine.

Experiences like that have left me with a newfound appreciation for clean public toilets—and the peculiar heroics of making it there in time.

Now, why am I telling you all this again? Well, it's not just for the chuckle. It's because this moment perfectly captures the wild unpredictability of IBS. It's terrifying, it's dramatic, and in hindsight, it's hilarious when you can look back on it and say, "I survived that".

But what about now? What's changed since then? A lot.

The Journey Beyond the Bus

Looking back, it's not just about that single moment of sheer panic; it's about the entire journey. It was actually around that time on the bus that I actually got a lot more serious about getting better. I've learned that managing IBS isn't about waiting for the next emergency but preventing it from happening in the first place. It took me years to stop seeing my gut as the enemy and start working with it instead of against it. And along the way, I picked up all the tricks in the book: rhythmic breathing, figuring out which foods trigger me (goodbye spicy noodles, we had a good run), and, most importantly, learning how to manage my stress before it managed me.

Don't get me wrong—I'm not saying it's been a flawless journey. There were still plenty of close calls, awkward moments, and times when I thought, *this is it*. But with each small victory (like not soiling myself in public), I learned something new.

For You, Fellow Traveler

So, if you've been reading this book wondering whether you're destined for a dramatic public incident like mine—fear not. While IBS can throw some serious challenges your way, you can dodge them with the right tools, mindset and attitude. You'll have days where it feels like a win just to get to the nearest bathroom, but you'll also have days where you forget all about your gut, and those days are the real victories.

If my journey can be summed up in one thought, it's this: IBS doesn't have to control you. You won't find me screaming on buses or making highway pit stops these days. Instead, I've learned to listen to my body, make adjustments, and most importantly, laugh at the absurdity of it all. Because if you can't find some humour in the chaos, what's the point?

Closing Thoughts

In the end, this book isn't just about my story—it's about yours too. If you've been on a similar journey, you know the ups and downs. And

I'm here to tell you, from one IBS warrior to another, that you've got this. The next time you feel that familiar twinge, remember: you're not alone, you're not a YouTube meme, and most importantly—there's always hope. And a bathroom nearby.

About the author

David is a teacher, writer, and advocate for gut health, based in the UK. Having taught in several countries, David has spent years navigating life with IBS, a condition that first appeared in his teens and was officially diagnosed in 2012. Despite years of frustration, it wasn't until 2016 that he began taking the first serious steps toward recovery. However, it would take another six years of trial, error, and self-reflection to finally achieve meaningful and lasting improvement.

Through thousands of hours spent researching books, videos, medical advice, and consulting doctors across multiple countries, David discovered that the most significant factor in overcoming IBS was... himself. By taking responsibility for his own habits and committing to consistent, holistic changes, he was able to reclaim his life from the grip of IBS.

Driven by a deep empathy for others struggling with the same condition, David wrote *The IBS Escape Plan* to save others from the years of frustration and pain he endured. The book isn't a subscription service or an expensive app—it's a call to action, a guide to taking accountability, and a step-by-step plan for real, sustainable change.

David understands all too well the daily challenges IBS sufferers face—from worrying about the nearest toilet to the dread of social gatherings or the agony of stomach pain. His passion for helping others stems from having been there himself and finding a way out. Through this book, he shares the realisation that the solutions to IBS aren't hidden in a product or prescription—they're within us, waiting to be unlocked. IBS can feel isolating, but you're not alone. This book is proof that with the right tools and mindset, real change is possible.

David's mission is simple: to help you find freedom from IBS and live a life of confidence and control.

To connect with David, follow him on social media @IBSEscapePlan.

youtube.com/@IBSEscapePlan

Appendix A

Scoring & Reflection

After writing, score each relationship from 1-10 based on how supportive and healthy it feels. Then, reflect on what steps you might take to address or improve the relationship.

Score	Definition
1-2	Very unhealthy: This relationship feels overwhelmingly negative. You feel drained, unsupported, or disrespected most of the time. Boundaries are often crossed.
3-4	Mostly negative: You often feel stressed, anxious, or unappreciated in this relationship. There are significant issues, and healthy boundaries are rarely respected.
Score	Definition
5-6	Neutral or mixed: This relationship has both positive and negative elements. There's some support, but it's inconsistent. Boundaries may be occasionally crossed.
7-8	Mostly positive: You generally feel supported and valued. There's a good balance of giving and receiving, with occasional minor conflicts or boundary issues.
9-10	Very healthy: This relationship is highly supportive and balanced. You feel uplifted and respected, and your boundaries are consistently honoured. Conflicts are rare and resolved constructively.

Evaluating Relationships Survey

Category	Prompts	Score (1-10)	Reflection/Next Steps
The Impact on Emotions	How positive are my feelings before I interact with this person? (e.g., excited vs. anxious)		Reflect on what makes interactions with this person either positive or stressful. How can you increase the positive feelings surrounding your time together?
	How do I feel during our time together? (e.g., relaxed, comfortable vs. stressed, uneasy)		If negative feelings dominate, consider whether there's a way to communicate or adjust your dynamics to make interactions more enjoyable.
	How do I feel after our interactions? (e.g., fulfilled, energised vs. drained, upset)		If you often feel drained afterwards, think about the cause and what steps you can take to manage or improve this outcome.
	Do I experience emotional ups and downs with this person, or is the relationship emotionally stable?		If there's emotional instability, reflect on whether setting clearer boundaries or addressing unresolved issues could help create a more balanced dynamic.

Category	Prompts	Score (1-10)	Reflection/Next Steps
Reciprocity Check	How well does this person support me when I need help (e.g., emotionally, practically)?		If support is lacking, what steps can you take to communicate your needs better? Or, consider whether this person is capable of offering the support you expect.
	How fairly do I support this person? Do I feel comfortable with the level of support I provide?		If the relationship feels unbalanced, think about how you can re-establish fairness and prevent over-giving or under-giving in a healthy way.
	How appreciated do I feel by this person for the support I offer?		If you feel unappreciated, reflect on whether you've communicated your feelings, and consider asking for more recognition of your contributions.
	Overall, how balanced is the give-and-take in this relationship?		If there's a mismatch in expectations or balance, think about whether the relationship needs renegotiation to better meet both of your needs.

Category	Prompts	Score (1-10)	Reflection/Next Steps
Boundaries Reflection	How often are my boundaries respected in this relationship?		If boundaries are often crossed, consider whether you need to be clearer about your limits or more assertive in maintaining them.
	How well do I assert my boundaries when they are challenged or crossed?		If you struggle with boundary enforcement, reflect on what might be holding you back and how you can improve your ability to communicate and protect your limits.
	How clearly have I communicated my boundaries in this relationship?		If boundaries feel unclear, reflect on how you can better communicate your limits moving forward, ensuring mutual understanding.
	How well do I respect this person's boundaries?		Reflect on how you can be more mindful of their boundaries and work on fostering mutual respect, which can enhance the relationship's health.

Category	Prompts	Score (1-10)	Reflection/Next Steps
Positives vs. Negatives	How would I rate this relationship's balance of positive versus negative interactions?		If the negatives outweigh the positives, think about ways to address or reduce recurring negative patterns and work on reinforcing the positive aspects.
	How frequently do conflicts or disagreements occur, and how well do we resolve them?		If conflicts are frequent and unresolved, reflect on conflict resolution techniques you could implement to ensure smoother communication and problem-solving.
	How constructive or damaging are our interactions when we disagree?		If disagreements are damaging, consider steps to improve how both of you approach and handle conflicts, perhaps through open discussion or setting ground rules for disagreements.
	How emotionally safe do I feel expressing my thoughts and feelings around this person?		If emotional safety is low, reflect on what specific behaviours or dynamics need to change for you to feel more comfortable sharing your feelings or setting boundaries.

Appendix B

*NOTE: Below are all the details surrounding what you can and can't eat. However, when you're on the go, I highly recommend using **ChatGPT** on your phone and it will guide you on whether or not you can eat something.*

So, the following table lists high-FODMAP foods and suitable low-FODMAP alternatives. Take your time with it and feel free to keep going back to it (as it does get confusing). Feel free to explore more sources for more detailed information or additional guidance.

Food Group	Foods to avoid	Suitable foods
Grains and starchy foods	• Amaranth • Barley • Freekah • Rye • Wheat (including bulgur wheat, couscous, semolina, sprouted wheat, wheat germ)	• Buckwheat flakes • Millet • Oats/oat bran • Polenta • Potato • Quinoa • Rice (white, brown, or basmati) • Sorghum
Bread	• Bagel • Brioche • Chapati • Ciabatta • Croissants • Focaccia • Garlic bread • Pitta bread • Rye bread • Wheat pizza base • All wheat bread and rolls (white, brown, granary, multigrain, soda bread)	• Wheat or gluten-free bread (such as those made from oats, rice, corn, potato, and tapioca flours) • Wheat-free or gluten-free bagels, ciabatta, naan, pitta bread and pizza bases • 100% sourdough spelt bread (Please make sure it is 100% spelt as many bakeries actually say it's spelt, but it's a mixed loaf.

Food Group	Foods to avoid	Suitable foods
Savoury biscuits and pastries	• Cream crackers • Crispbreads • Rye crispbreads • Shop-bought pastry (puff, flake and shortcrust made from wheat flour, including pie, quiche and pasties) • Spelt crackers • Water biscuits • Wheat crackers	• Oatcakes (check ingredients of flavoured varieties) • Plain or ready-salted crisps • Wheat-free or gluten-free pastry
Pasta and noodles	• All fresh and dry wheat-based pasta • Gnocchi • Spelt pasta • Udon noodles • Wheat noodles	• Buckwheat (soba) noodles and pasta • Quinoa pasta • Rice noodles and pasta • Wheat-free or gluten-free pasta
Breakfast cereals	• Honey flavoured cereals • Wheat, spelt or bran-based cereals (Weetabix, shredded wheat, bran flakes, all-bran, cheerios, muesli)	• Crisped rice cereal (e.g. rice krispies) • Gluten free cornflakes • Porridge and some oat-based cereals (check cereals for other high FODMAP ingredients) • Rolled oats

Food Group	Foods to avoid	Suitable foods
Flours and baking	• Almond flour • Amaranth flour • Barley flour • Coconut flour • Lupin flour • Rye flour • Soya flour • Spelt flour (excluding 100% sourdough spelt bread) • All wheat flour (white, wholemeal, plain, self-raising)	• Baking powder • Bicarbonate of soda • Buckwheat flour • Cornflour • Cream of tartar • Maize flour • Millet flour • Oat flour • Polenta • Potato flour/starch • Pounded yam • Quinoa flour • Rice flour • Sorghum flour • Tapioca flour/starch • Teff flour • Wheat-free or gluten-free flour (excluding those listed in foods to avoid, e.g., lupin flour)
Cakes, sweet biscuits, cakes, pastry	• Any made from wheat or other high FODMAP flour (such as wheat-based biscuits - digestive, shortbread, etc., wheat-based cake, wheat-based sweet pastries)	• Coconut macaroons • Flapjacks (check for honey as an ingredient) • Flourless cakes or cakes made with low FODMAP flour • Meringues • Oat-based biscuits

Food Group	Foods to avoid	Suitable foods
Fruit (fresh, dried, juice) Limit to three portions per day Limit portion size of suitable foods to one portion per snack/meal. The (1) represents the number or amount allowed per sitting. Generally, the portion size = 80g fresh fruit, 13g dried fruit, 100ml fruit juice	• Apple • Apricot • Blackberries • Boysenberries • Cherries • Figs • Goji berries • Lychee • Mango	• Banana (1 firm, not ripe) • Blueberry • Breadfruit (1) • Cantaloupe melon (1 slice) • Carambola/starfruit (1) • Clementine (2) • Coconut (dried, shredded) (30g) • Coconut (fresh) (64g) • Cranberries (small bowl)

Food Group	Foods to avoid	Suitable foods
Fruit (fresh, dried, juice): Limit to three portions per day. Stick to one portion per snack/meal: 80g fresh fruit, 13g dried fruit, or 100ml fruit juice. The (1) represents the number or amount allowed per sitting.	•Nectarine •Peach •Pear •Persimmon (sharon fruit) •Plum •Pomegranate •Prunes •Tinned fruit in apple or pear juice •Tinned guava •Watermelon •Fruit juices (except cranberry juice) •Most dried fruits (some allowed in small serving sizes; see moderate foods table below)	•Dates (dried, pitted) (5) (excluding medjool dates) •Dragonfruit (1) •Durian (1) •Grapes (10) •Guava (ripe, peeled) (2) •Honeydew melon (1 slice) •Kiwifruit (2) •Lemon (juice of 1) •Lime (juice of 1) •Mandarin (1-2) •Orange (1) •Papaya/paw paw (1 slice) •Pineapple (140g) •Raspberries (58g, small bowl) •Rhubarb •Starfruit (1)

Food Group	Foods to avoid	Suitable foods
Vegetables	• Artichoke and artichoke hearts (tinned) • Asparagus • Beans and pulses (including broad beans, black-eyed peas, butter beans, lentils, baked beans, kidney beans, and split peas) • Beetroot (raw) • Broccoli (stalks) • Brussel sprouts • Butternut squash • Savoy cabbage • Cauliflower • Celery • Chicory root	• Alfalfa • Aubergine • Bamboo shoots • Beansprouts • Beetroot (pickled in vinegar) • Bok choy • Cabbage (red, white) • Carrot • Cassava • Celeriac • Chard/swiss chard • Chicory (leaves) • Fresh chilli • Chives • Choy sum • Cucumber • Endive
Vegetables	• Garlic • Karela • Leek (white part) • Mange tout • Mushrooms (except oyster mushrooms) • Onion • Peas • Pumpkin	• Fennel (leaves) • Ginger • Green beans • Kale • Leek leaves (green part only) • Lettuce • Okra • Olives (green, black)

Food Group	Foods to avoid	Suitable foods
Vegetables	• Savoy cabbage • Shallots • Spring onion (white part) • Sugar snap peas	• Green bell pepper • Pak Choy • Parsnip • PlantainPotato • Radish • Rocket • Seaweed nori • Spinach • Spring onion (green part) • Swede • Sweetcorn (canned and drained) • Sweetcorn (fresh from cob, up to ½ cob) • Turnip • Water chestnut • Yam
Milk and dairy-free alternatives: Check labels for added FODMAPs like apple juice, FOS, or inulin.	• Buttermilk • Condensed milk • Evaporated milk • Lactose • Milk powder • Milk solids • Milkshakes • Skimmed milk powder • Soya milk	• Coconut milk (less than 125ml) • Hemp milk (less than 125ml) • Lactose-free milk • Lactose-free yoghurt (check ingredients), yoghurt made with suitable milk alternative

Food Group	Foods to avoid	Suitable foods
Milk and dairy-free alternatives: Check labels for added FODMAPs like apple juice, FOS, or inulin.	• Whole, skimmed, semi-skimmed milk (cows) • Yoghurts (all including Greek, drinking and diet varieties, fromage frais, soya yoghurt)	• Nut milk (almond, macadamia)Oat milk (less than 120ml) • Rice milk (less than 200ml) *Please ensure all alternative milk are calcium-enriched.*
Cheese	• Cottage cheese • Cream cheese • Halloumi • Low-fat soft cheese • Processed cheese, cheese slices, reduced-fat cheese • Quark • Ricotta	• Blue • Brie • Camembert • Cheddar • Edam • Feta • Goats cheese • Mozzarella, parmesan, pecorino, swiss cheese
Other dairies See note for milk	• Custard • Malted milk drinks (for example horlicks, bournvita, Ovaltine, milo, options, drinking chocolate) • Soya custard • Soya ice cream	• Butter • Crème fraiche • Cream • Ice cream (up to 1 scoop) (check for high FODMAP flavours) • Lactose-free ice cream • Sour cream • Sorbet (made from low FODMAP fruits, check ingredients)

Food Group	Foods to avoid	Suitable foods
Nuts and seeds	• Cashews • Pistachio	• Seeds • Most nuts (except almonds and hazelnuts, which are suitable only in limited amounts)
Drinks Take 6-8 glasses (1.5 - 2 litres) of fluid per day.	• Chai tea • Chamomile tea • Chicory (camp coffee) • Coconut water • Dandelion tea • Fennel tea • Oolong tea *Avoid teas with high FODMAP additives, such as apple, pear, or stone fruits (e.g., peaches).*	• Black coffee (or with suitable milk/milk alternative) • Black tea • Green tea • Lemon tea • Orange peel tea • Peppermint tea • Rooibos tea
Alcohol	• Dessert wine • Fruit ciders • Port • Rum • Sherry	• Most alcoholic drinks: Wine, beers, vodka, gin, whiskey

Food Group	Foods to avoid	Suitable foods
Sugars and sweeteners	• Fructose-based sweeteners such as glucose-fructose syrup, fructose syrup, high fructose corn syrup • Honey • Isomalt • Jams made from high-FODMAP fruits • Sweeteners ending in 'ol': Erythritol, Maltitol, Mannitol, Sorbitol, Xylitol • Sweeteners may be added to mints, chewing gum, chocolate, sweets or drinks	• Acesulfame k • Aspartame • Canderel • Dextrose • Glucose • Glucose syrup • Golden syrup • Jam/marmalade (made from suitable fruits in the suitable section above) (check for high FODMAP sweeteners) • Maple syrup • Saccharin • Stevia • Sucralose • Sugar (brown, white, caster, icing etc.) • Treacle

Food Group	Foods to avoid	Suitable foods
Herbs, spices, flavourings, condiments and other ingredients to look out for.	• Casein • Dried onion – powder, puree, extract or dried • Fructo-oligosaccharides (FOS) • Garlic – powder, puree, extract, salt • Inulin • Lactose • Milk fat • Milk protein • Milk solids or milk powder • Most pre-made pasta sauces • Pickled onions • Vegetable pickles/relish	• Arrowroot • Baking powder, bicarbonate of soda, cream of tartar • Buckwheat flour • Cider vinegar • Cornflour • Garlic infused oil • Herbs and spices such as chilli, dried herbs, vinegar, pepper and salt • Maize flour • Mayonnaise (check ingredients for added garlic/onion) • Millet flour • Mint sauce/jelly • Miso paste
Herbs, spices, flavourings, condiments and other ingredients to look out for.		• MSG • Polenta • Soy sauce • Spring onion (green part) • Tomato sauce (up to 26g/1 tbsp) • Worcestershire sauce • Yeast

Appendix C

Moderate FODMAP containing foods

Some foods higher in FODMAPs, as identified by reputable resources[1] [2] [3], can be included during the restriction phase but only in small amounts and one food at a time. The following tables detail these 'moderate' FODMAP servings and the suitable amounts. You do not need to include these foods but can choose to if it is helpful.

---

1. Fody Foods. *How Much Can I Eat?*. Accessed November 22, 2024. https://www.fodyfoods.com/blogs/news/how-much-can-i-eat?utm_source=chatgpt.com

2. Monash University. *How to Avoid FODMAP Stacking*. Accessed November 22, 2024. https://www.monashfodmap.com/blog/how-avoid-fodmap-stacking/

3. Monash University. *Monash University FODMAP Diet App*. Accessed November 22, 2024. https://www.monashfodmap.com

Food Group	Food	Quantity allowed
Dairy	Halloumi	up to 2 slices
	Quark	up to 2 tbsp
	Reduced-fat cheese/ cottage cheese/ cream cheese/ low-fat cheese	up to 2 tbsp
	Ricotta	up to 2 tbsp
	Soya yoghurt	up to 2 tbsp
	Yoghurt	up to 1 tbsp
Fruit	Avocado	up to 40g
	Cherries	2 (20g)
	Currants/raisins	1 tbsp
	Dried banana	15 chips (30g)
	Dried cranberries	1 tbsp
	Grapefruit	½ medium (104g)
	Lychees	3 pieces (50g)
	Pomegranate	45g
	Tamarind	4 pieces (8g)
	Strawberries	6 strawberries (75g)
Nuts/seeds	Almonds	10 nuts
	Hazelnuts	10 nuts
	Chia seeds	up to 24g/2 tbsp

Food Group	Food	Quantity allowed
Vegetables	Broccoli (head)	75g (when raw)
	Butternut squash	up to 45g
	Celery	10g ¼ stick
	Courgettes	up to 75g
	Mange tout	up to 5 pods (16g)
	Peas	up to 1 tbsp (15g)
	Sundried tomatoes	up to 4 pieces
	Sweet potato	up to 75g
	Sweetcorn	up to 3 tbsp (40g) or ½ cob
	Fennel bulb	¼ bulb
	Fresh tomato	up to 60g
	Red, yellow or orange bell pepper	up to 47g

Flavourings	Oyster sauce	up to 1 tbsp
	Tamarind paste	up to 1/2 tbsp
	Balsamic vinegar	up to 1 tbsp

Snacks	Plain corn cakes	up to 1 cake
	Plain rice cakes	up to 4 cakes
	Milk chocolate	up to 20g
	White chocolate	up to 25g
	Dark chocolate	Up to 30g

Appendix D

Symptom Recording Template

Below is an example of how to document your symptoms during the reintroduction phase of the low FODMAP diet. Use this format in your symptom notebook to track your progress.

Important: If you experience symptoms on Day 1, stop testing that food and move on to the next one.

Food used: Garlic (Fructan)

Day	Quantity	Symptoms
1	¼ clove	None
2	½ clove	None
3	¾ clove	Abdominal Pain & Bloating

Food used: White bread (Fructan)

Day	Quantity	Symptoms
1	1 slice	Diarrhoea
2	-	-
3	-	-

Food used: Avocado (Sorbitol)

Day	Quantity	Symptoms
1	¼	None
2	½	None
3	¾	Abdominal Pain & Bloating

Appendix E

You can choose one food from each table below:

Fructan - Grain Foods

	Day 1	Day 2	Day 3
Wheat Pasta	5 tbsp (cooked)	10 tbsp (cooked)	15 tbsp (cooked)
Breakfast cereal (Bran Flakes or Weetabix)	1 tbsp or 1 biscuit	2 tbsp or 2 biscuits	3 tbsp or 3 biscuits
Bread, wheat, white or wholemeal	1 slice	2 slices	3 slices

Fructan - Fruit and Vegetables

	Day 1	Day 2	Day 3
Brussel sprouts	3 sprouts	4 sprouts	5 sprouts
Leek	½ leek	1 leek	1 ½ leeks
Grapefruit	½ medium	1 medium	1 large
Raisins	1 ½ tbsp	2 tbsp	3 tbsp

Fructan - Garlic

	Day 1	Day 2	Day 3
Garlic	¼ clove	½ clove	¾ clove

Fructan - Onion

	Day 1	Day 2	Day 3
Onion, any	1 tbsp	2 tbsp	3 tbsp

Fructan + GOS

	Day 1	Day 2	Day 3
Bread, wheat, wholegrain	1 ½ slice	2 slices	3 slices
Beetroot, fresh	3 slices	4 slices	6 slices
Cashew nuts	10 nuts	20 nuts	30 nuts
Pistachio nuts	15 nuts	30 nuts	40 nuts
Peas, frozen	40g	80g	120g

Appendix F

Lactose

	Day 1	Day 2	Day 3
Cow's milk	120ml	250ml	375ml
Yoghurt, plain	125g	250g	375g

Sorbitol

	Day 1	Day 2	Day 3
Corn on the Cob	½	1	1½
Avocado	¼	½	¾
Blackberries	2-3 berries	5 berries	10 berries
Peach	¼ medium	½ medium	1 medium

Mannitol

	Day 1	Day 2	Day 3
Button mushroom	½ small	2 small	4 small
Cauliflower	60g	120g	180g
Celery	25g	50g	75g
Sweet potato	100g	200g	300g

Fructose

	Day 1	Day 2	Day 3
Asparagus	1 spear	2 spears	5 spears
Honey	1 tsp	2 tsp	3 tsp
Mango	¼ mango	½ mango	¾ mango

GOS (Galacto-Oligosaccharides)

	Day 1	Day 2	Day 3
Almonds	15 nuts	20 nuts	30 nuts
Canned chickpeas, rinsed	80g	160g	240g
Butter beans	40g	80g	120g
Silken tofu	45g	90g	180g

If you prefer to try out different high-FODMAP foods, please find more examples of the five main FODMAP groups you'll be testing in the table below.

Fructose (Monosaccharide)	Lactose (Disaccharide)
• Apples • Pears • Mango • Honey • High-fructose corn syrup • Watermelon • Agave syrup • Asparagus • Sugar snap peas • Cherries • Grapes • Pineapple • Lychee • Blackberries • Coconut water • Papaya • Raisins • Persimmon • Tomatoes • Sugarcane	• Cow's milk • Yoghurt • Soft cheeses (e.g., ricotta, cottage cheese) • Ice cream • Custard • Goat's milk • Cream cheese • Buttermilk • Pudding • Sour cream • Ricotta • Mozzarella • Butter (in large amounts) • Feta cheese • Whey protein • Cream • Kefir • Processed cheeses • Dairy-based sauces (e.g., cheese sauce
Fructans (Oligosaccharide)	**Galacto-Oligosaccharides (GOS) (Oligosaccharide)**
• Garlic • Onions • Wheat (bread, pasta) • Barley • Rye • Artichokes • Leeks • Cabbage • Asparagus • Chicory root • Broccoli • Beets • Brussels sprouts • Fennel • Shallots • Radicchio • Okra • Pistachios • Cashews • Inulin (added to some processed foods)	• Chickpeas • Lentils • Black beans • Kidney beans • Soybeans • Pistachios • Cashews • Green peas • Baked beans • Split peas • Navy beans • Lima beans • Hummus • Fava beans • Puy lentils • Black-eyed peas • Edamame • Snow peas • Sugar snap peas • Soy milk

Polyols (including Sorbitol and Mannitol)	
•Avocado	•Sweet corn
•Cauliflower	•Lychee
•Mushrooms	•Cherries
•Blackberries	•Apricots
•Apples	•Watermelon
•Pears	•Bell peppers
•Nectarines	•Prunes
•Sugar-free gum (with sorbitol or mannitol)	•Pineapple
	•Coconut
•Stone fruits (e.g., plums, peaches)	•Carrots

Printed in Great Britain
by Amazon

59898543R00288